Celebrating the Cycle

Guiding Your Daughter into Womanhood

Celebrating the Cycle Books

Celebrating the Cycle ~ Guiding Your Daughter into Womanhood

Second Edition

ISBN: 978-0-9762535-4-9
LCCN: 2008910021

Published by Celebrating the Cycle Books
701 South 2nd Street
Fairfield, IA 52556
http://www.celebratingthecycle.com
email: mariezenack@gmail.com

Book Interior by Marie Zenack & Christina Wadsworth.

Cover Art by Christina Wadsworth.

Printed and Distributed by Lightning Source.
http://www.lightningsource.com

Zenack, Marie.
    Celebrating the Cycle ~ Guiding Your Daughter into Womanhood /
    Marie Zenack. -- 2nd ed.

ISBN: 978-0-9762535-4-9

Acknowledgements

I thank my husband, Nathan, for supporting me in the writing of this book; my granddaughters, for inspiring me to write quickly, in order to be ready when their passage into womanhood arrives; my children and their spouses, for introducing me to family-centered birth and creative parenting; my daughter, Christina Wadsworth, for her soft and passionate art work; Stephen Kelley and Amanda Cousins, for technical support; my friends and family, for attentive editing; and the mothers of Fairfield, Iowa, whose concern for their daughters planted the seeds of this book in my heart.

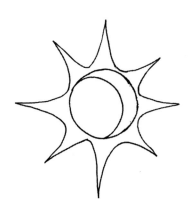

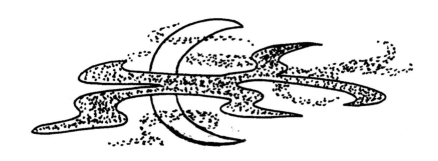

Dedicated to my mother,
and her mother,
and all mothers.

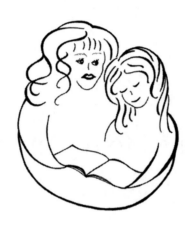

Contents

Illustrations

Stories and Legends

Poems

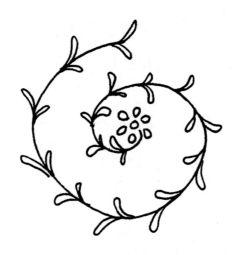

Making the Best Use of This Book

This book is a step-by-step guide for you as a mother to use as you lead your daughter through her passage into womanhood. If you read it yourself before reading it with your daughter, you will know which parts are right for your daughter, and when.

The first section, "Understanding the Cycle," can be read with your daughter before she begins menstruation. You may notice physical changes transforming your little girl into a woman: underarm hair, pubic hair, developing breasts. Your daughter may have questions about the changes happening in her body. Or she may seem more silent than usual—pondering and wondering. At times, unexplained mood swings may surprise you both. These are some signs it is time to read through the first section of this book together.

Please do read *with* your daughter. How many of us remember the lonely experience of trying to learn about our bodies from a book handed to us by an embarrassed mother? May we all heal those old memories as we walk the road again with our own daughters!

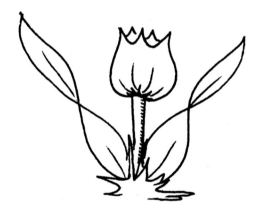

You may want to read the first section together with your daughter several times, leaving a few weeks between each reading. Even more important than the information are the emotions that may arise during the weeks and months after the first reading. Take time to discuss feelings. Take time to read again.

The second section, "Creating the Celebration," helps you as a mother plan a ceremony to honor your daughter's passage into womanhood. Ceremonies that mark an important change in a person's life are called rituals. Weddings, graduation ceremonies, and baby showers are some familiar rituals. In our community of women we refer to menstruation as our "moon-time." We therefore call the ritual marking a woman's first menstruation a first moon-time ritual. A moon-time ritual can make this time easier and more meaningful. It comforts the young woman, letting her know her feelings are natural and have been shared by women throughout time. It focuses the attention of the community on the young woman's needs at this time in her life. And it instructs the young woman about what her family and society expect of her now that she is entering womanhood. (1) Knowing that a nurturing gathering of supportive women is waiting to receive your daughter will allow you both to feel more secure during those weeks and months before her first bleed. It is ideal to read "Creating the Celebration" before your daughter begins her first bleed. However, even if your daughter has already begun menstruating, a moon-time ritual will be a joyful experience for everyone. In our community we have known some 19-year-old big sisters who demanded a moon-time ritual when their younger sisters received theirs!

When your daughter's first moon-time (menstruation) arrives, read the first section "Understanding the Cycle" one more time together. You will have her attention now. And there will be questions that did not come up before. Then call together your community of women to participate in the ritual you have planned. Let other women support and nurture you both at this tender time.

Don't worry if some of the women are embarrassed by the idea of a moon-time ritual. Their feelings will be healed as they join in the honoring of your daughter. And please don't put off your daughter's ritual because she is shy and doesn't want to tell anyone "she has started." This is her moment. I recommend helping her to face it and feel good about it. Surround her with women she loves and who love her. You may be surprised, especially if you have never attended a moon-time ritual, at the healing and joy that accompany such a gathering. Have your daughter's ritual, if possible, within the first few days or weeks after her first bleed. One mother, who had her community of women ready, was able to have her daughter's first moon-time ritual during her daughter's very first bleed.

Only you will know when it is time to read the third and last section of this book, "Sexuality and Birth," with your daughter. Remember, the longer you put it off, the more likely it is that her peers or her school will give your daughter this special information. She may get accurate information that way, or she may not. In any case, she will miss your spirit as she absorbs this new concept of herself as a sexual being. Notice her interests. Is she looking at herself in mirrors? Is she more aware of boys? Does she have questions about love or babies? If so, it is probably time to read "Sexuality and Birth" together. Many mothers say they like to give their daughters time to get used to menstruation before reading "Sexuality and Birth." But some daughters are excited and interested in everything having to do with babies. Trust your mothering instincts. There is no need to give information for which your daughter is not ready. Neither is there a need to withhold information that your daughter wants or needs. Don't worry if your daughter does not absorb all the information in the first reading. There is plenty of time for second readings.

When you have gone through all the material together, you may want to leave this book out where you and your daughter can easily refer to it. When questions arise, you can reread sections together. Or your daughter may want to ponder the book alone. These pages are meant to make information easily available whenever the teachable moment arrives. Perhaps your daughter is one of the lucky ones and has been getting clear explanations about sex and babies since she was in diapers. Still, you may find, as I did, that a loving discussion of sexuality and birth with a daughter who is herself becoming a sexual being is different and more challenging for us as moms. At such a time, a step-by-step guide can be helpful.

May we all heal ourselves,
as we learn anew with our daughters.

Section One

Understanding the Cycle

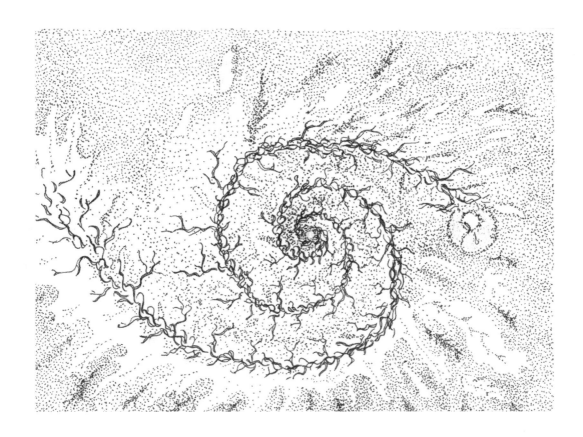

Life moves and evolves in cycles.

Planets and stars revolve and spin.

Galaxies turn round their centers.

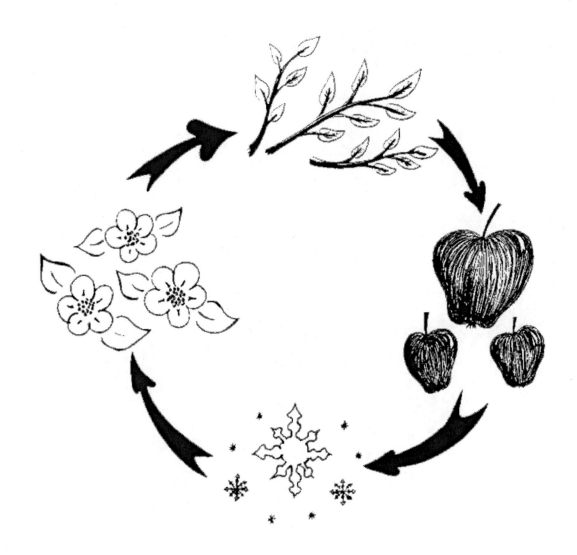

Seasons give way to seasons: The abundance of summer finds fulfillment in autumn, which is followed by the deep sleep of winter, before awakening to the new life of spring, and moving back to abundance.

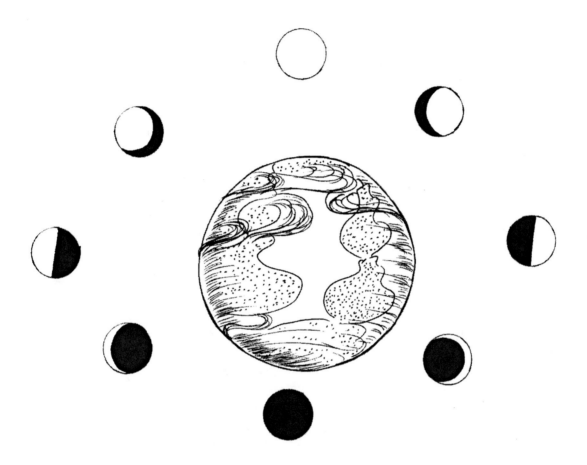

Grandmother Moon shines in her fullness, then retreats slowly into hiding, before returning to fullness.

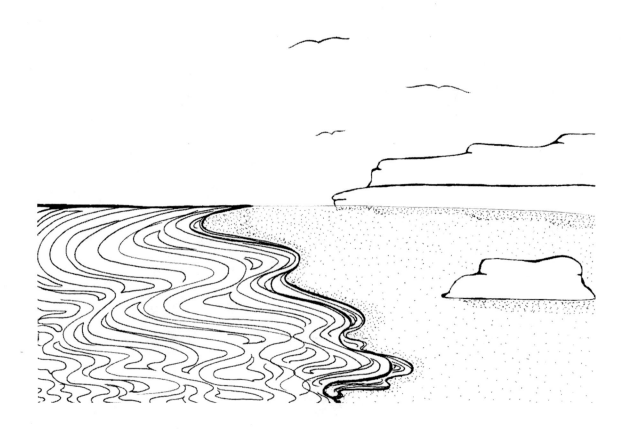

Circling around the Earth, Grandmother Moon pulls and releases the oceans, causing the tides, high and low.

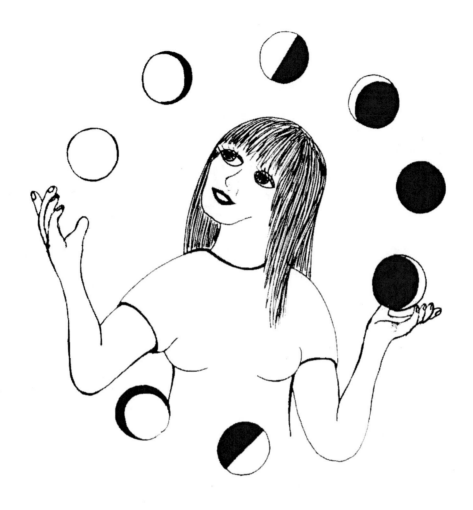

The waxing (growing larger)
and waning (becoming smaller)
of Grandmother Moon
stir the cycles within us.
Cycles of creativity,

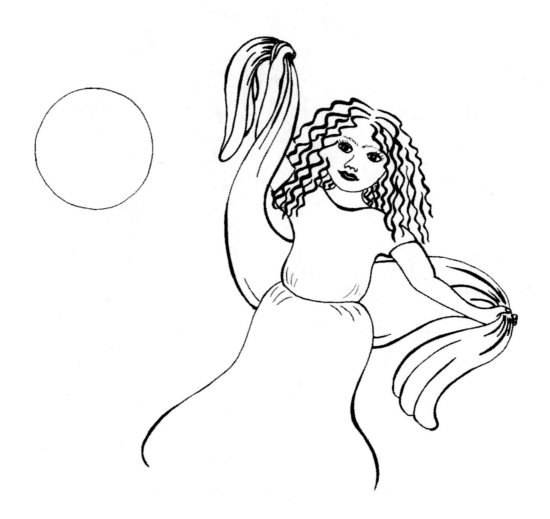

energy,

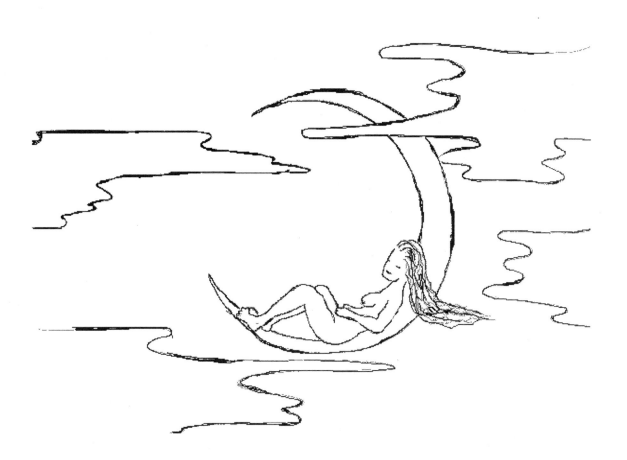

... and fertility.

Our cycle of fertility means that someday we can become moms. Our cycle begins in our brain, which sets the cycle in motion by sending hormones to the rest of the body.

Hormones are minute substances manufactured by certain glands in our bodies. Hormones travel through the bloodstream and play an important role in activating many of the body's functions.

Although there has been much scientific study of hormones, many of their functions are still unknown. However, we know the hormones are being sent from our brain because our bodies begin to go through changes.

Our breasts grow bigger. Hair grows under our arms. Hair grows between our legs. (Hair between our legs is called pubic hair.)

These changes are the beginning of becoming a woman.

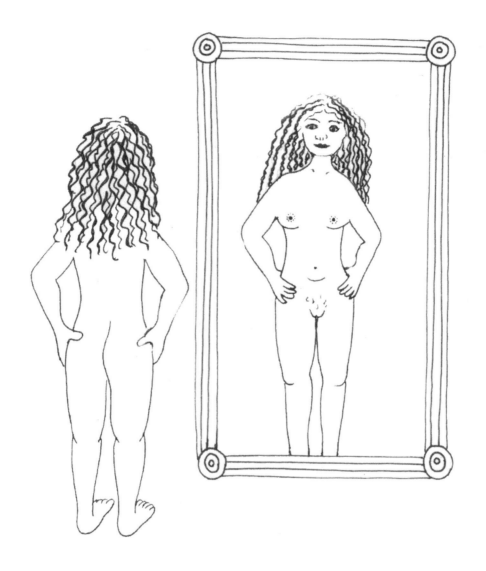

Even if the changes seem unfamiliar to you now,
you will soon begin to enjoy
the beauty and confidence
womanhood brings to you.

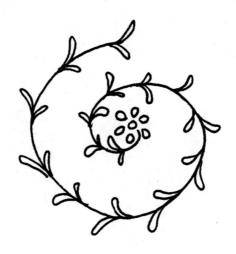

A Woman's Organs of Fertility

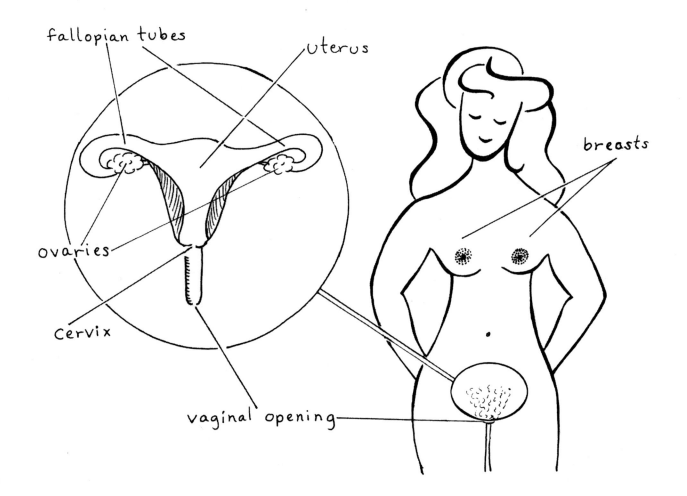

Here is a drawing of our organs of fertility. We have drawn them outside the body so we can see them, even though they are mostly inside. We have two ovaries, which are glands about the size of unshelled almonds (about one to one-and-a-half inches). Each of our ovaries contains about 200,000 little unripe follicles, which are tiny rings of cells. Each follicle has a tiny unripe egg, called an ovum, inside. (You can see the ovum without a microscope, but just barely.) The ova (plural of ovum) were present in your body even before you were born, while you were still growing inside your mother.

Someday, if you become a mom yourself, one of these tiny ova will grow and develop into your own baby.

We have two fallopian tubes, which are soft and flexible tubes leading from the ovaries to the uterus, or womb. When an ovum is released from one of the ovaries, it travels along one of the fallopian tubes towards the uterus.

The uterus is where a baby grows and develops inside its mother. Inside the uterus is a lining, called the endometrium, which is a soft bed that can nourish and support the growth of a baby.

The cervix is the opening of the uterus. The cervix connects to the vagina, which is a soft and flexible canal leading to the outside of the body. You can find the outside opening of the vagina between your legs, between the hole where you pass urine (the urethra) and the hole where you pass bowel movements (the anus).

This is why it is important, when wiping with toilet paper after using the toilet, to wipe from front to back. Wiping from back to front may drag bacteria from the anus to the vagina or urethra, causing infection.

Folds of skin, called labia, surround and protect both the urethra and the vaginal opening. (2)

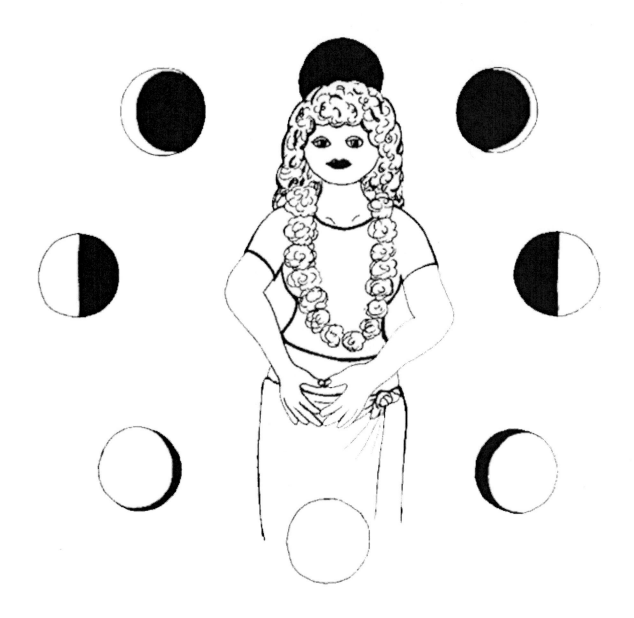

Put your hands pointing downward on your lower abdomen with your thumbs on your navel (your belly button). Let your index fingers meet at the bottom. Your little fingers will be over your ovaries. Your index fingers will be over the top of the uterus. The bottom of the uterus is the cervix, the opening. It is deep inside your body, opening into the top of the vagina. (3)

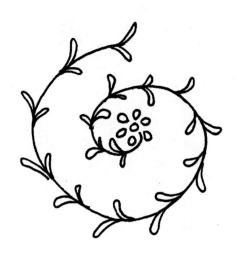

A Woman's Cycle of Fertility

When fertility begins, hormones from the brain cause the ovaries to begin ripening some of those little unripe ova which have been waiting in our ovaries since before we were born.

Hormones also cause the cervix to begin making a certain kind of moisture: cervical mucus.

Cervical mucus is produced by the cervix as the ova are maturing in the ovaries. The mucus flows down the vagina and we notice it outside the vaginal opening, between our legs. It is not enough moisture to soak our clothes. We may mistake it for perspiration or an infection, but it is the natural mucus produced by our cervix as the ova mature in our ovaries.

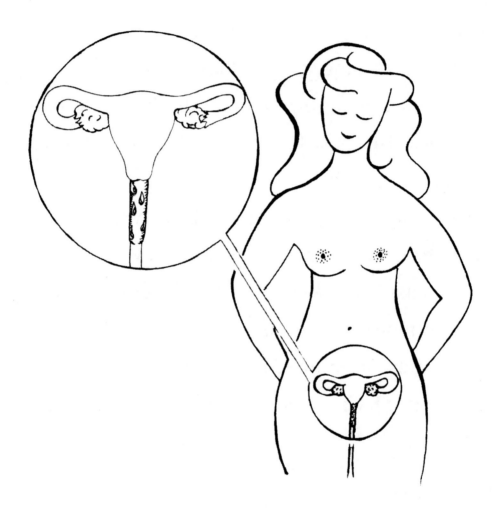

You may notice the mucus for a few days, only to have it disappear and return in a few more days or weeks. It takes time for the first ova to mature.

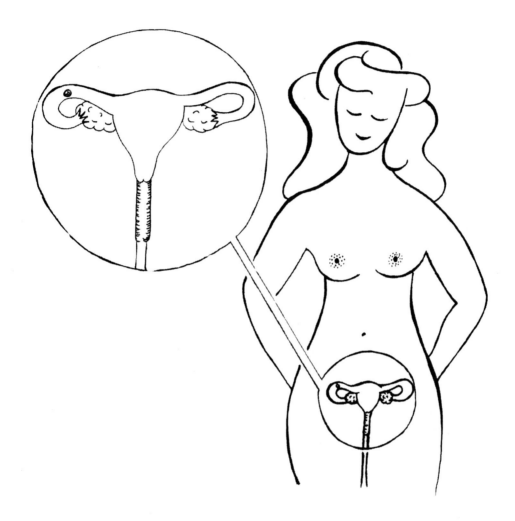

However, eventually, in response to the hormones, one of the maturing ova is released into a fallopian tube.

This is called ovulation.

The ovum travels along the
fallopian tube toward the uterus.

An ovum lives for less than 24 hours
before it disintegrates and is absorbed by the body.

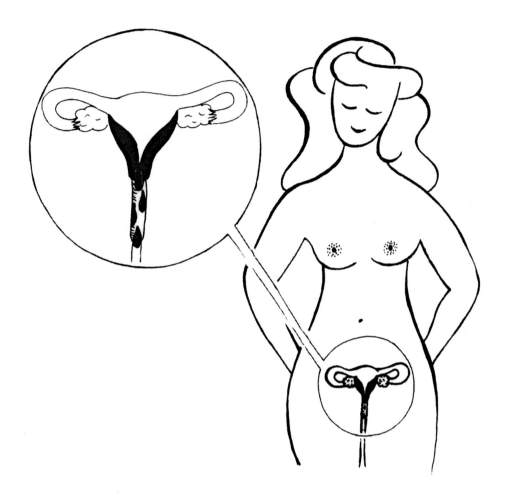

About two weeks after ovulation, our bodies realize that the lining of the uterus is not needed to nourish a baby this cycle.

The lining is then shed in what is called "menstruation." Menstruation is also referred to as "our period" or "our moon-time."

During our period, we see and feel blood outside the vaginal opening between our legs. The menstrual flow is actually the lining of the uterus. But since the tissue of the uterine lining contains blood, menstruation is a bloody flow.

We usually notice the bleeding first on our underpants or on the toilet paper when we use the toilet. Menstruation contains the nutrients that would have held and nourished a baby if this were the time in our lives to become moms.

As soon as the lining of the uterus (endometrium) is shed with menstruation, another lining begins to grow.

That is the nature of a cycle:

One ends. Another begins. (2)

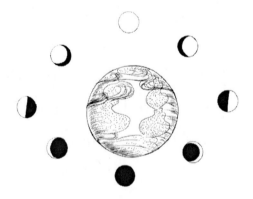

The Bra

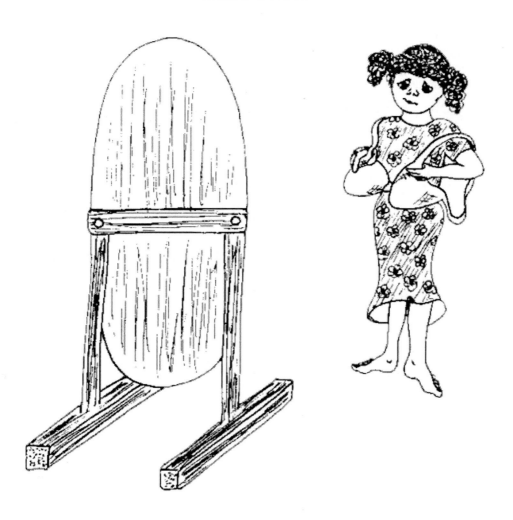

These are times of change. You may feel shy, as if everyone were looking at you. And it may be true. Everyone may be looking at you. But if they are, it is only because you are beautiful and full of life at this time.

So feel good about your changing body.

Your growing breasts will someday, if you become a mom, be able to make milk for your baby.

These are also times when retailers will begin to advertise things to you—like bras. You don't need to wear a bra unless you are more comfortable wearing one.

A camisole may be an alternative; some of them have shelf bras built in. Our society expects women to cover their breasts. So we might begin to feel uncomfortable if our breasts show through our clothing.

However, bras that alter our shape, push our breasts up, have underwires, or cut off our circulation are associated with health concerns for women. This is a good time to begin to learn what not to buy.

The problem with bras is that they can block the circulation of the lymph system. So if you wear a bra, it should be loose enough not to leave lines on your skin when you take it off.

And, according to research on women's health, the more time spent without a bra, the better. You can take off your bra when lounging at home and, of course, while sleeping. Plenty of time spent bra-less is an important way to learn what is natural and comfortable for your breasts. (4)

Hormones and Emotions

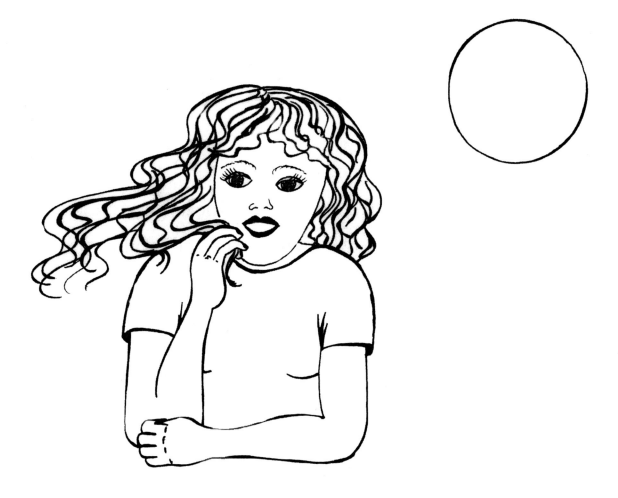

During each phase of our cycle,

a different hormone is active in our bodies.

Hormones affect how we feel.

The hormone estrogen is most active during the wet time of our cycle.

Estrogen can make us feel self-confident, out-going, creative, and full of energy.

We may feel less need to sleep, because the hormone adrenaline, which causes excitement, is also high in our bodies at this time.

Our wet time is really our power time. It is a time to start new projects or to finish old ones.

Like Grandmother Moon in her fullness, we may feel assertive, friendly, and much more loving.

If we are aware of our cycle phases, we can be more productive and more able to harness our energy to fulfill our personal goals. (2)

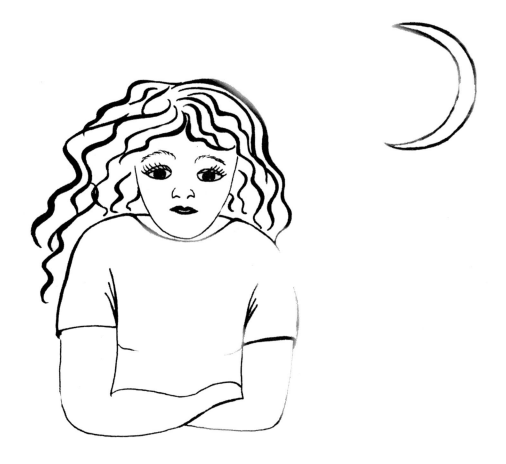

After the ovum is released from our ovary, the hormone progesterone becomes active in our bodies. Progesterone can make us feel somewhat deflated compared to our wet time.

We may feel like being quiet and inward.

During menstruation, our bleeding time, both estrogen and progesterone are low in our bodies.

Just as Grandmother Moon covers her face and withdraws at the end of her cycle, we may feel like being alone at the end of ours.

We may be more sensitive. (2)

We may be more intuitive.

Intuition refers to our ability to directly know the truth without a complicated reasoning process.

If we understand and follow the natural inward and outward flow of energies in our bodies, with each cycle we will begin to intuit more and more of our own personal direction and truth. (5)

Learning from our Ancestors

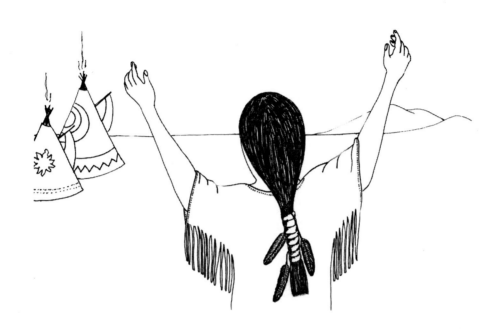

In previous centuries, some tribes of Native American women went into the moon lodge, a dwelling apart from the activities of daily living, during the time of their moon-time bleeding.

In the moon lodge women could rest and renew themselves and "call vision" for their people.

Calling vision referred to seeking inner direction from the spiritual realm. It was believed that the veil between ordinary life and the spiritual mysteries of creation was thin at the time of bleeding.

Because of the thinning of this veil, a woman in her moon-time was believed to be especially intuitive.

When the women came out of the moon lodge, they were asked what truth they had seen for their people. In this way, the people were led and protected.

According to Brook Medicine Eagle, a Native American Earth wisdom teacher, the most important contribution a woman can make to her culture, even today, is to live in harmony with her moon-time cycle. (5)

The Moon-Time

We may bleed (menstruate) for three to five days, sometimes longer. The last one or two days may be light bleeding or just spotting.

And women usually menstruate every 28 to 30 days, or about once a month. If you are just beginning your fertility, your cycles may be irregular. You may have a bleed and then not have another for six months.

Or your cycles may be regular from the beginning.

But however long or short, regular or irregular, your cycles may be, you will notice a time of out-going, active energy, as well as a time of inward, quiet energy.

The waxing and waning aspect of creative energy is the unique contribution of women to culture.

A woman learns from her own body that all things have their time.

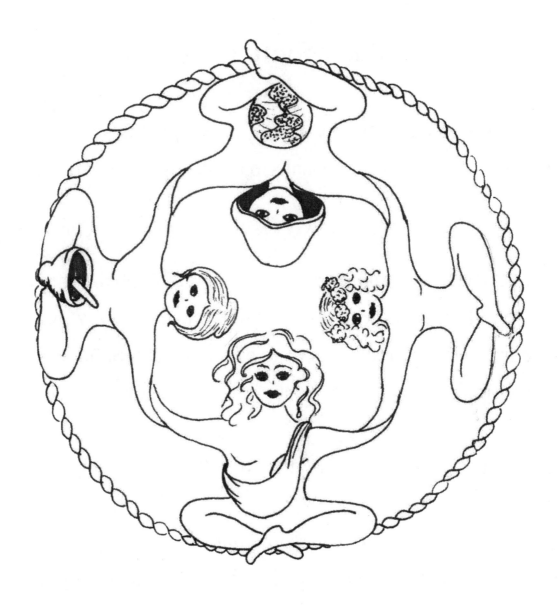

Everything ends.
And every ending
carries within it
the seeds of a new beginning.

Women Artists

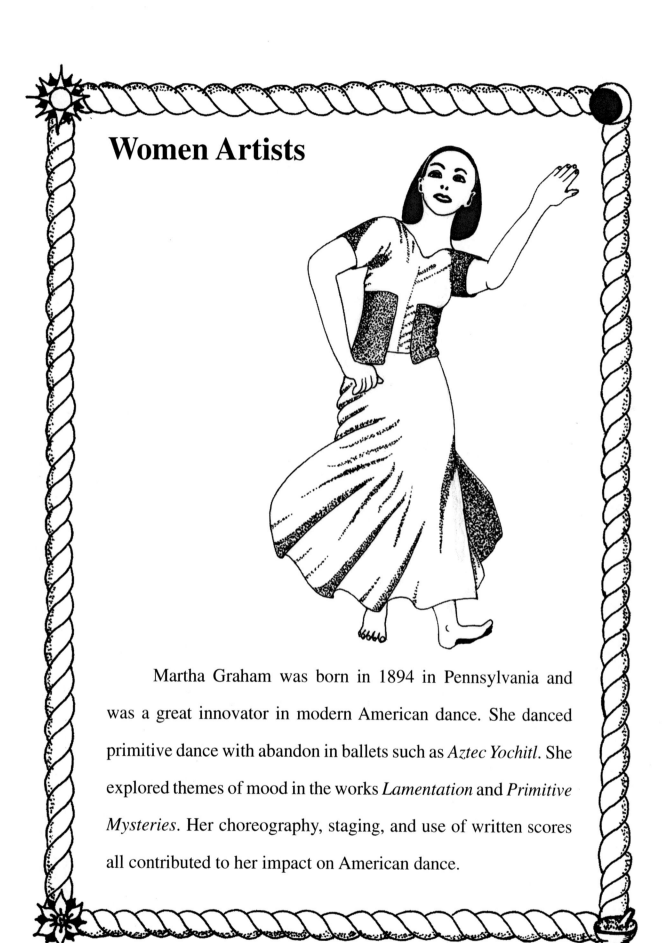

Martha Graham was born in 1894 in Pennsylvania and was a great innovator in modern American dance. She danced primitive dance with abandon in ballets such as *Aztec Yochitl*. She explored themes of mood in the works *Lamentation* and *Primitive Mysteries*. Her choreography, staging, and use of written scores all contributed to her impact on American dance.

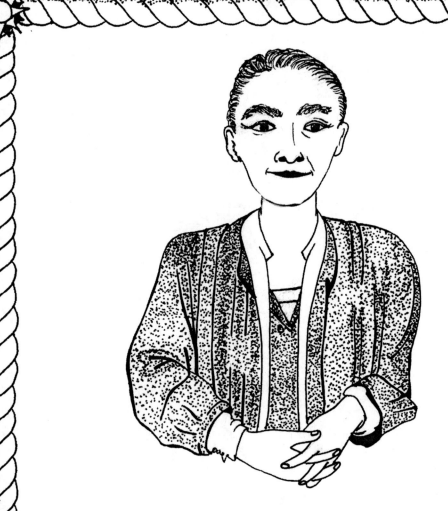

Born in Wisconsin in 1887, Georgia O'Keefe was a well-known American artist. Her early work was formal and abstract, using natural forms such as flowers and animal skulls. Later she painted rural scenes that included barns and Mexican-Indian buildings. Georgia worked into her nineties. She was elected to the American Academy of Arts and Letters in 1963 and to the American Academy of Arts and Sciences in 1969. She is famous for her original style.

Charting the Moon-Time

May 2005

Sun	Mon	Tue	Wed	Thu	Fri	Sat
1	2	3	4	5	6	7
Red	**Red**	**Red**	**Spots**			
8	9	10	11	12	13	14
15	16	17	18	19	20	21
22	23	24	25	26	27	28
29	30	31				

Charting our cycles, beginning even with our very first menstruation, is a way to keep in touch with our bodies, our feelings, and our health. Many women like to keep a calendar or a notebook that is only for charting their moon-time cycle.

You can mark the days of bleeding in some way, such as coloring the calendar day red or writing the word "bleeding," or "red." On some days, you will feel nothing and see nothing outside the vagina. You can leave the calendar blank on those days.

May 2005

Sun	Mon	Tue	Wed	Thu	Fri	Sat
1 **Red**	2 **Red**	3 **Red**	4 **Spots**	5	6	7
8	9	10	11	12 ◊	13 ◊	14
15	16	17	18	19	20	21
22	23	24	25	26	27	28
29	30	31				

But on other days you will feel, or maybe see, *something* outside the vagina. You can write down on that calendar day what you feel and what you see. At first you may notice only pasty or sticky mucus or just a feeling of wetness. You can write "pasty," or draw raindrops to indicate wetness on these days.

May 2005

Sun	Mon	Tue	Wed	Thu	Fri	Sat
1 **Red**	2 **Red**	3 **Red**	4 **Spots**	5	6	7
8	9	10	11	12	13	14
15	16	17	18	19	20	21
22	23	24	25	26	27	28
29	30	31				

As your cycles become more regular, you may begin to notice a slippery feeling, or a clear, elastic mucus. This mucus is not a sign of illness or uncleanliness. It is a sign that an ovum is ripening in your ovaries. You can color the raindrops dark to indicate the slippery wetness.

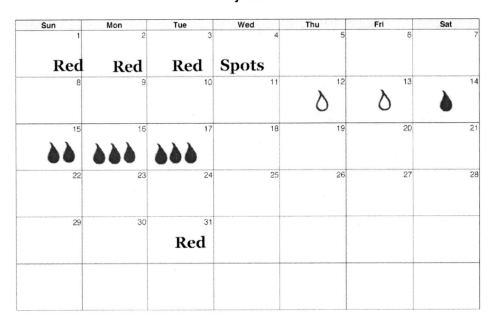

May 2005

Sun	Mon	Tue	Wed	Thu	Fri	Sat
1 **Red**	2 **Red**	3 **Red**	4 **Spots**	5	6	7
8	9	10	11	12	13	14
15	16	17	18	19	20	21
22	23	24	25	26	27	28
29	30	31 **Red**				

After a few wet or slippery days, the moisture may disappear or return to sticky or pasty. When it does, you will know that an ovum has probably been released from one of your ovaries. The release of the ovum from the ovary is called ovulation. Once ovulation has occurred, your next bleed will come in about two weeks. If you pay attention for a few cycles, you will soon be able to predict your bleeds in advance, even if your cycles are irregular.

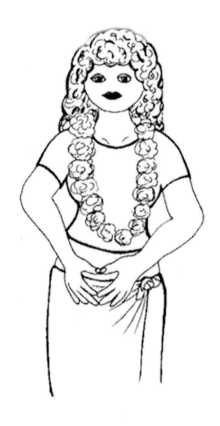

Notice when the slippery mucus becomes sticky, or perhaps disappears. When it does, count ahead about two weeks on your calendar to predict your time of bleeding.

You will become quite accurate about these predictions. The time between ovulation and your next bleed will be between 11 and 16 days. You will learn your unique time after a few cycles of charting. (6)

You may notice a slight twinge of pain near the ovaries at the end of your wet time. This is probably ovulation—the release of the ovum from the follicle.

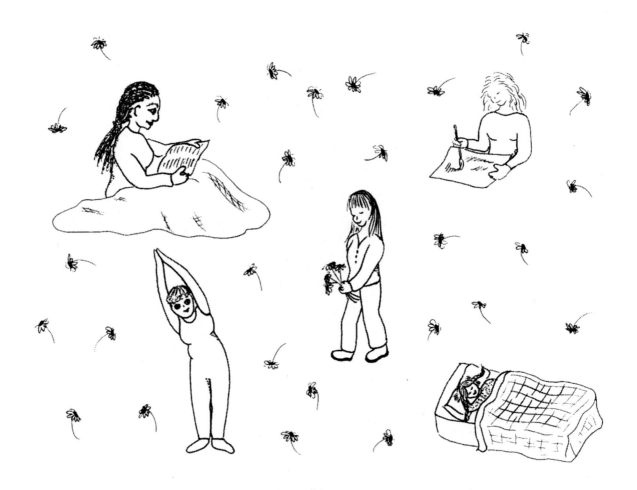

Once you predict the time of your next bleed, you can start planning your quiet time. Perhaps there is a book you have been meaning to read, or a walk in the woods you would enjoy. You can begin to look forward to your own very personal time of retreat.

Even if you have to go to school or work, you may be able to reserve a little time for yourself for resting and renewal. Many women find that they are able to accomplish much more during their entire cycle if they allow a time of retreat during menstruation.

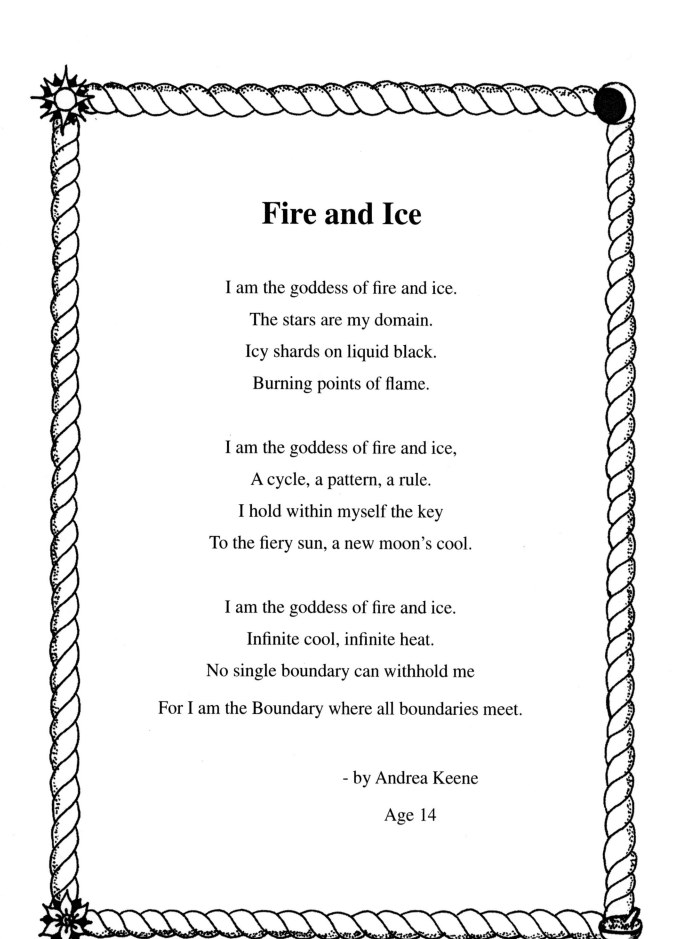

Fire and Ice

I am the goddess of fire and ice.

The stars are my domain.

Icy shards on liquid black.

Burning points of flame.

I am the goddess of fire and ice,

A cycle, a pattern, a rule.

I hold within myself the key

To the fiery sun, a new moon's cool.

I am the goddess of fire and ice.

Infinite cool, infinite heat.

No single boundary can withhold me

For I am the Boundary where all boundaries meet.

- by Andrea Keene

Age 14

Ancient Moon-time Charts

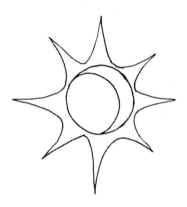

The first markings on stone ever discovered are believed by anthropologists to be moon-time markings—women keeping track of their menstrual cycles and the relationship of their menstrual cycles to the cycles of the moon. These moon-time charts eventually developed into full lunar calendars—complicated records of events based on the cycles of the moon.(7) In a lunar calendar, a month begins with each new moon. The new moon is the day the moon begins to grow bright again, after being completely dark. The length of a lunar month is the length of time between two new-moon days: 29 to 30 days.

Our word mathematics, or math, comes from the word, mathesis, or ma thesis, which means mother wisdom. It originally referred to astronomy and astrology. The first astronomers and astrologers were called "Wise Mothers," even if they were men. The name "Wise Mothers" acknowledged that the sciences of the skies were invented by women as they charted their menstrual cycles and the cycles of the moon and other heavenly bodies. (7) It is fun to realize that women pilots and astronauts are following in the footsteps of thousands of centuries of women who invented the charting of the skies. This beautiful and ancient lunar notation was identified on the walls of the famous caves at Lascaux, in France.

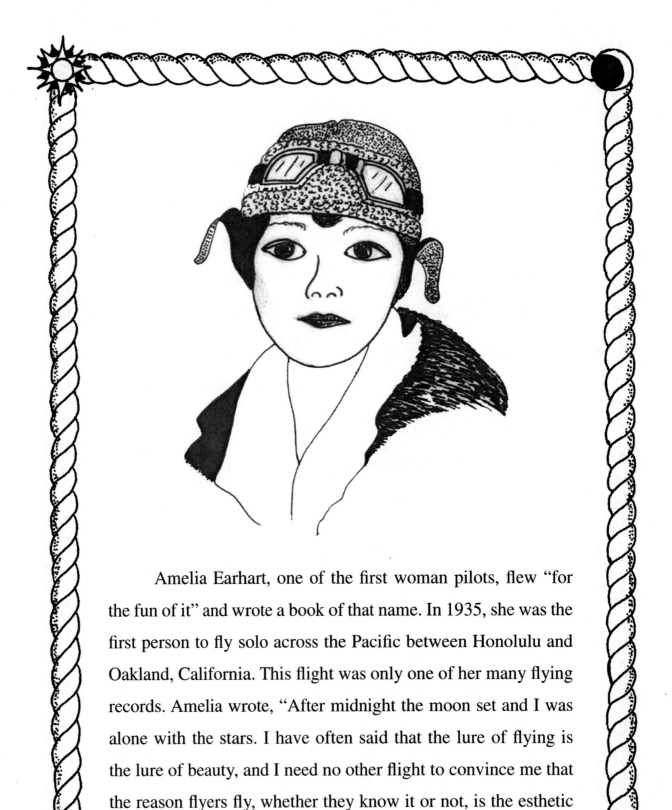

Amelia Earhart, one of the first woman pilots, flew "for the fun of it" and wrote a book of that name. In 1935, she was the first person to fly solo across the Pacific between Honolulu and Oakland, California. This flight was only one of her many flying records. Amelia wrote, "After midnight the moon set and I was alone with the stars. I have often said that the lure of flying is the lure of beauty, and I need no other flight to convince me that the reason flyers fly, whether they know it or not, is the esthetic appeal of flying."

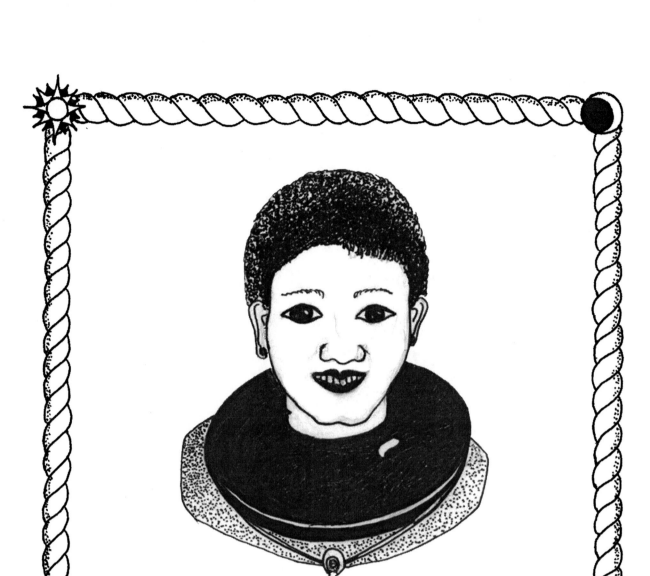

Dr. Mae Jemison was aboard the space shuttle Endeavor in 1992. In addition to having been an astronaut, she is a chemical engineer, scientist, physician, and teacher. Mae is also versed in African and African-American Studies and is trained in dance and choreography. She has always followed her dreams, undaunted by a lack of role models in her fields of endeavor and roadblocks to the advancement of women and minorities.

Health

Now is a good time to begin to take care of your health, and your moon-time cycle is a measure of your health. If you feel weak or sick during your bleeding time, or if you have discomfort before or during, or if you are not enjoying your moon-time in any way, your overall health may need some attention.

There are many natural herbal, homeopathic, or nutritional formulas to help us maintain balance and health. A warm herbal tea made from nettle and raspberry leaf is an excellent tonic for women of all ages. It is important to remember that drugs or artificial hormones do not really balance or heal our bodies. They only cover up problems temporarily, while causing long-term, serious health problems themselves. (8)

So you see you have many good reasons to begin now to learn about health and natural healing. There are health reference books listed at the back of this book that will get you started exploring health.

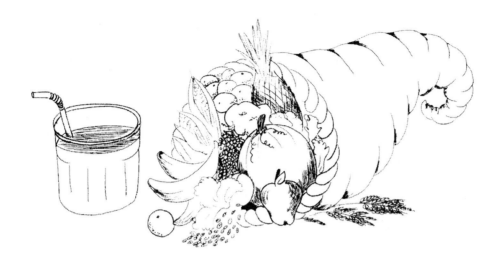

Eating and eliminating form another of nature's cycles. Young bodies need plenty of nutrition on a regular basis, preferably from whole foods grown without chemicals. In addition to causing disease, nutritional deficiencies can leave us open to unhealthy cravings for "junk food," alcohol, or drugs. (9)

Drinking plenty of pure water and eating plenty of fiber, such as is found in fresh fruits and vegetables, will support regular bowel movements, which are important for overall health and hormonal balance. According to many schools of natural healing, consuming ice-cold foods and drinks causes weakness and menstrual discomfort. (10)

Sleep

Rest and activity form yet another of nature's cycles. Sleep is nature's way of renewing and maintaining balance—physically, emotionally, and spiritually. Teenagers need about 9.5 hours of sleep each night. It is thought that sleep requirements increase for teens because the hormones that are essential for maturing bodies are released mainly during sleep. Yet studies show that most teenagers only get about 7.4 hours of sleep a night. This is not enough for a teen to be healthy. (11)

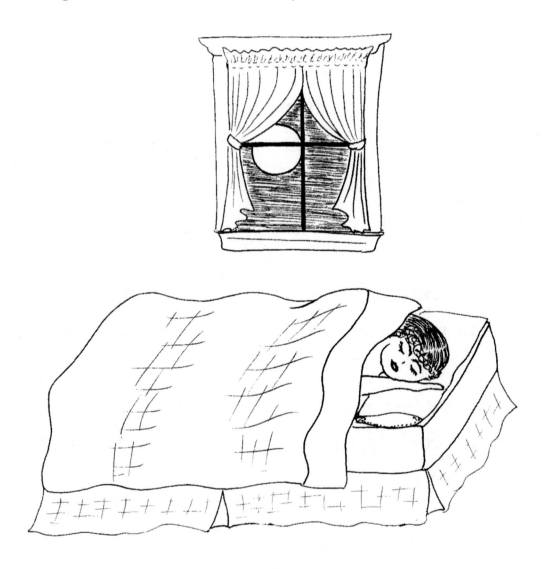

Lack of sleep leaves us confused and undirected, open to the chaotic influences of others who are also sleep-deprived. Deep and regular sleep keeps us in close contact with our own inner knowing and moves us steadily toward the accomplishment of our goals.

Intuition

Asking inwardly for direction before going to bed at night and waiting for the answer in the early morning hours is a practice used by women throughout the centuries to develop clearer intuition. (12) If you wish to try this simple practice, wait until you are in bed, quiet and relaxed, just before falling asleep. Make your request or ask your question of the Divine within you. Fall asleep naturally. In the morning, do not jump up immediately. Wait for a few minutes, expectantly but not anxiously, to see if some intuitive "knowing" comes to you. Do not be discouraged if it doesn't. It takes time to develop intuition. And the answer may come later on in some quiet moment, when you least expect it. Answers from the Indwelling Divine fill us with peace and security. We know with confidence how to proceed. Or we know with confidence we are protected and guided.

Beauty

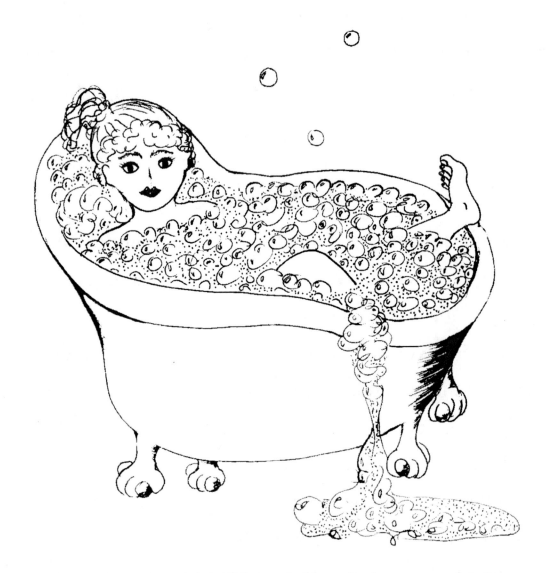

Beauty is a multi-billion dollar industry, which means makeup and skin care companies will be looking for your attention. Some of these "beauty" products contain substances that may actually cause skin problems over time. Reading labels on whatever we buy is an important skill. Simple and natural is safest and best.

Cleanliness is the simple basis of all beauty. Now that you are growing up, society expects you to know how to care for your body. Shampooing and bathing, washing feet and underarms, and changing clothes, especially blouses and socks, keep us feeling and smelling fresh.

Whatever we use to wash our bodies should have a pH of 5.5, which is close to the pH of our skin. Alkaline products (above pH 5.5) strip the protective coating from the skin. This invisible coating is made of oil and sweat. The loss of its protective coating can cause the skin to go wild in the production of oil, furiously trying to replace the protective layer that was lost. This excess oil can clog the pores and actually cause skin blemishes. Alkaline bubble bath products can irritate the tender skin of the urethra and cause pain during urination.

You can check the pH of products if you are interested in doing so. Inexpensive pH testing kits are available at drug stores and pet stores. Soap, whether in liquid form or a bar, is always too alkaline. The liquid washes or gels are usually the correct pH to protect the skin.

If you want to use a deodorant, please read the label carefully. It is important that it not contain aluminum, which is associated with many health concerns. Potassium alum, on the other hand, is considered safe.

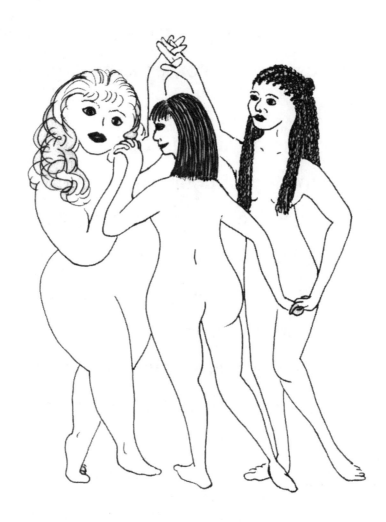

Throughout history, a woman's physical beauty has been the subject of art. However, the idea of what is beautiful keeps changing! No matter what the ideal of physical beauty may be at any time, it is women's inner beauty that truly inspires and leads the culture. As you put your attention on what society calls beautiful, remember to let your inner, and very individual, beauty shine forth.

Caring for Our Skin

Blemished skin can be treated with raw, unfiltered apple cider vinegar, which has many healing properties and is pH 5.5. Splash or dab it on blemished skin after bathing. If you continue to be troubled with skin blemishes, consider strengthening your liver, which is your body's cleansing organ. Milk thistle is an herb widely known for supporting liver function. The extract of milk thistle is stronger and more effective than the ground herb powder and is available in any health food store or food co-op.

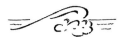

Caring for Our Clothes

During your moon-time you may find that the hot water of a bath or shower causes you to bleed a little more. Try drying between your legs with toilet paper after your bath or shower to avoid staining your towel. Stains can usually be removed with cold water and detergent. Use hydrogen peroxide for more stubborn stains.

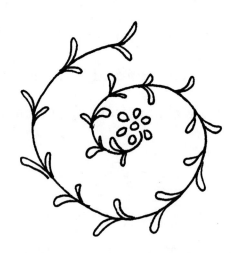

Harmonizing our Cycles
With the Cycles of Grandmother Moon

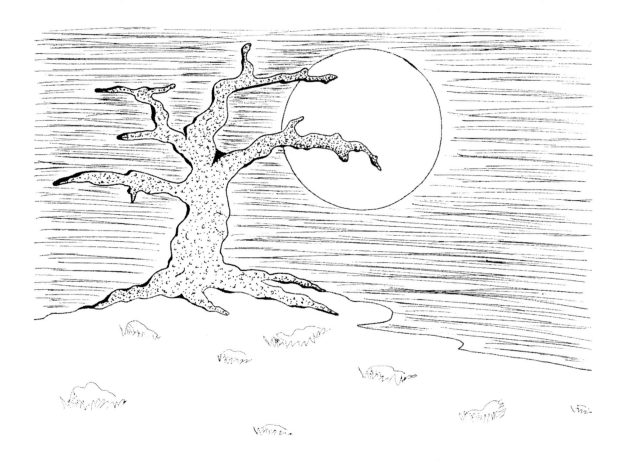

According to some traditions, women who live under Grandmother Moon's light will tend to ovulate on the full moon and menstruate on the new moon. In our community of women, we have found that cycles are easier and more harmonious if they follow the cycles of Grandmother Moon in this way. When menstruation falls on the new moon, bleeding does not seem as heavy. Ovulation on the full moon seems most natural.

Because we are surrounded by so much artificial light, even while sleeping, it can be a challenge to get in tune with the moon's cycles. Research shows that women's cycles normalize when artificial light is eliminated while sleeping. Artificial light while sleeping appears to interfere with the production of melatonin, which is a hormone associated with ovarian activity. (14)

Women report being able to gradually harmonize their cycles with the cycles of Grandmother Moon by sleeping in total darkness, except for one or two nights at the time of the full moon. If you want to try sleeping in darkness, make some dark shades for your bedroom windows and make sure there is no light of any kind from your clock radio, from under your door, etc.

For one night during the full moon, open your shades and sleep in the moon's light. If this is not possible, get a night light and use it only during the night of the full moon. You may have to continue this practice for some months, so be patient. You may enjoy seeing your cycles gradually respond to Grandmother Moon's light.

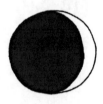

Menstrual Pads

The beginning of each menstruation is signaled by a wet feeling at the vaginal opening that you will soon learn to recognize. Just before your period begins you may also notice physical sensations that are caused by the hormonal changes in your body. Some women notice tender breasts. Others feel a slight heaviness in the lower back. Still others feel abdominal cramping. These sensations are different for everyone, but learning to recognize them will allow you to know when your period is about to begin.

Because the flow of menstruation is heavy enough to soak through our clothes, it is important to learn to care for ourselves and our clothing. Many products are available to absorb our menstrual flow and make our moon-time comfortable. You can buy 100% cotton pads, called sanitary napkins or menstrual pads. They are very comfortable to wear. Make sure to carry a few of these pads, and maybe a spare pair of underpants, in your purse or back pack in case you begin your moon-time away from home. If you begin your period at school, the school nurse or secretary will usually have menstrual pads to give you. Peel off the sticky paper on the bottom side, and place the sticky side of the pad on your panties, between the legs. It will absorb the menstrual flow.

Menstrual Pad

Pad with "Wings"

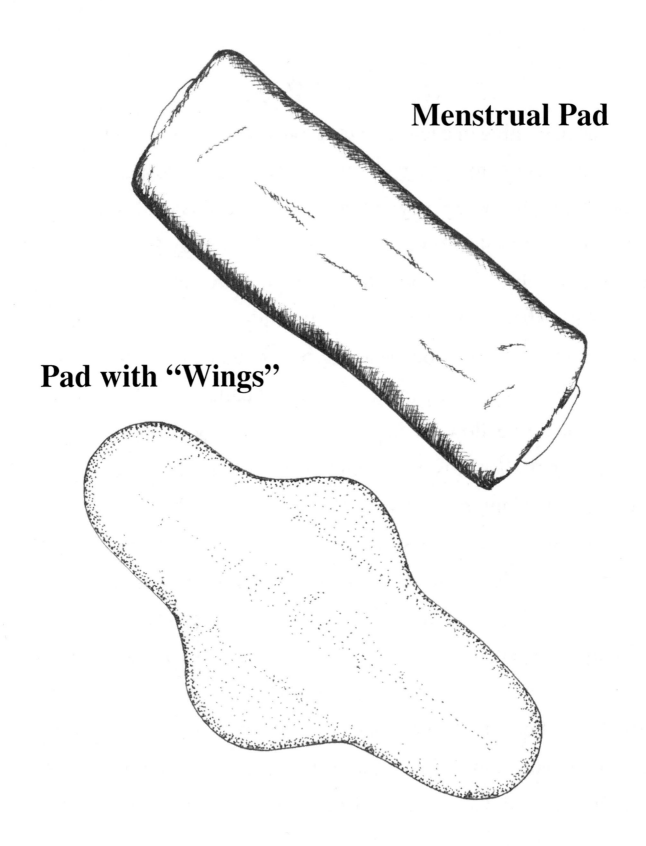

Pattern for Reusable Pads

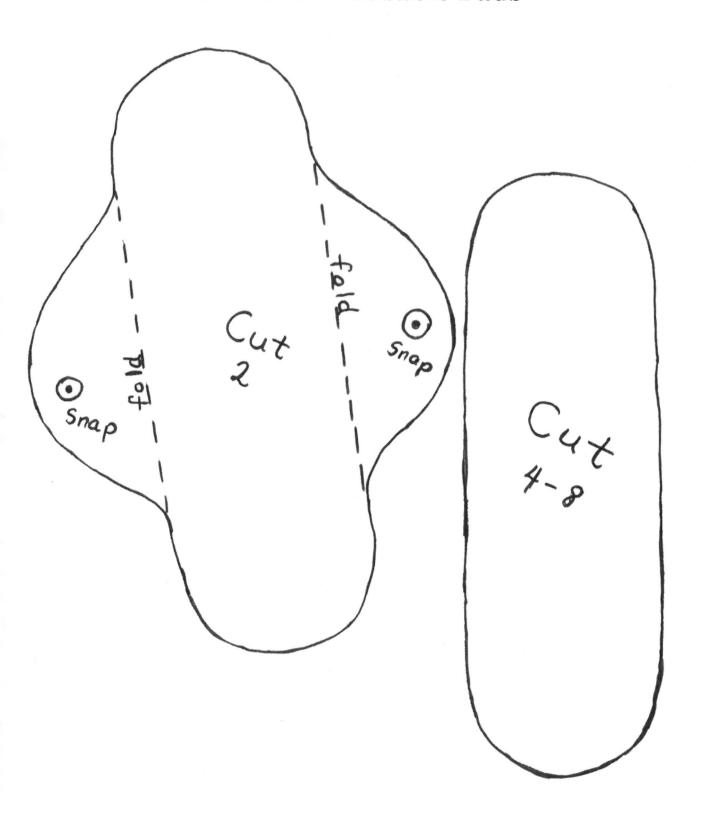

69

In about two hours, when you go to the bathroom again, you can take off the pad, fold it in half with the used side to the inside, wrap it in toilet paper or a paper towel, and throw it in the trash.

Usually public bathrooms have little trash cans inside the stalls that are meant for used pads. Or you can discard the used pad in the regular trash can. But don't try to flush it down the toilet, because it won't flush!

Washable Menstrual Pads

Many women enjoy using washable, reusable, cotton menstrual pads, which can be easily made or purchased over the Internet. Reusable pads must be soaked in cold water after each use, before washing them in warm, soapy water. You can make your own reusable pads using the pattern on the previous page.

Use absorbant cotton such as diaper cotton. Stack four to eight layers between a winged piece on top and bottom. Using the zigzag stitch on your machine, sew all around the outer edges. Add snaps. Wings are folded around the crotch of the underpants and snapped together underneath. Make 10 to 15 pads for your convenience. Make pads of different thicknesses for days of light or heavy flow.

Tampons

Tampons are little plugs of absorbent material that can be inserted into the vagina to absorb the menstrual flow before it leaves the vagina. They allow us more freedom during our moon-time but are more difficult to learn to use than pads. And they raise serious health concerns.

Tampon

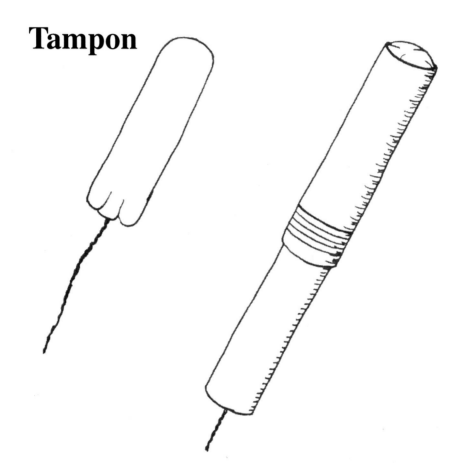

Tampon with Applicator

The natural secretions of the vagina are constantly cleaning the vagina and making the growth of bacteria unlikely. The tampon, however, is not a natural part of this cleaning process.

Soon after a tampon is inserted, bacteria will begin to grow on the tampon. Bacteria, like all living things, eat and digest something and then excrete waste products. The waste products excreted by the bacteria are absorbed by the vagina. There have been cases of women becoming seriously ill and even dying from absorption of the waste products on a tampon. This "disease" is called toxic shock syndrome. The symptoms of toxic shock syndrome are: fever, vomiting, sunburn-like rash, diarrhea, muscle aches, dizziness, and confusion. (15)

If you begin to feel uncomfortable in any way while wearing a tampon, remove it immediately. Better yet, don't use tampons at all. If you decide to use tampons and want to reduce the risk, you can buy the unbleached organic cotton variety. Bleached cotton or synthetic tampons have been shown to contain dioxins, contaminates associated with serious health problems. (15) Always remove a tampon in two hours or less, and NEVER sleep with them.

Another concern with tampons is their effect on the body's natural flow of energy. According to many schools of natural healing, the body's energy naturally flows down during menstruation. (10) Many women experience that a tampon blocks the downward flow of energy and causes abdominal discomfort and cramping, which they do not experience when they use pads. Some women have even begun to call tampons "crampons!"

Tampons and the Hymen

The hymen is a thin membrane that partially closes off the vagina. It is about an inch and a half inside the vagina, and sometimes makes inserting a tampon difficult. There is an opening in the hymen to allow us to have our moon-time bleeding. The size of the opening varies from woman to woman. The membrane of the hymen is flexible, however, and it is usually possible to insert a small tampon comfortably if the menstrual flow is heavy enough to provide lubrication.

Read the directions on the tampon box. Some tampons come with a cardboard or plastic applicator, which is supposed to make it easier to insert the tampon. When inserting a tampon, point the front of the tampon back toward your spine. Don't point it up toward your heart, because your vagina doesn't go that way. And don't use force when inserting a tampon. If it proves difficult, wait. It may get easier with time because the membrane of the hymen stretches with growth and ordinary exercise such as biking and running. (16)

Tampons have a string that hangs outside the vaginal opening. The string makes the tampon easy to remove. Don't try to flush tampons, however, because over time they can cause the plumbing to back up. Just wrap them in paper and put them in the trash.

Inserting a Tampon

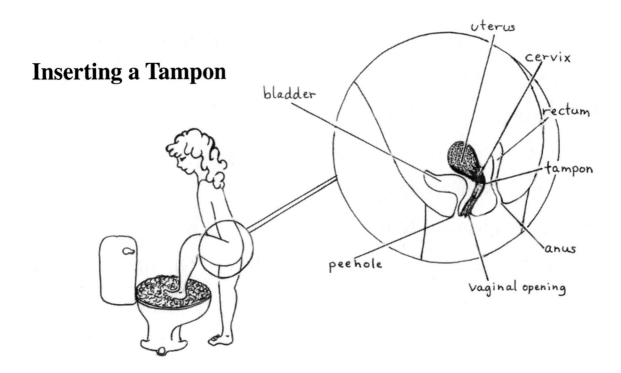

bladder
uterus
cervix
rectum
tampon
anus
peehole
vaginal opening

If you want to go swimming during your moon-time, a tampon allows you to do so. And the cool water will probably slow the bleeding for a while. However, according to many schools of traditional medicine, swimming in cool water during menstruation cools the internal organs, which over time causes menstrual discomfort and cramping. And swimming during menstruation increases the chance of infection in the uterus because the cervix is open during menstruation. If you decide to swim during your days of bleeding, be sure to remove the tampon after swimming. And take time for a warm bath or a warm heating pad over your lower abdomen after swimming.

Whenever possible, consider using menstrual pads instead of tampons. Get to know the downward flow of energy during your moon-time and enjoy taking your ancient and sacred time of retreat. Doing so will renew your energy and creativity each cycle.

Giving Back to Mother Earth

In the days of the Native American moon lodge, menstrual blood was considered sacred. In gratitude for the life-giving power of a woman's body, indigenous women sat on moss or straw, which absorbed their menstrual flow, and returned their life-giving blood to fertilize Mother Earth. This practice created a great circle of giving and receiving of fertility. (5)

Even today, many women enjoy watering their flowers with the soaking water from their re-usable cotton menstrual pads.

Your Personal Wisdom Path

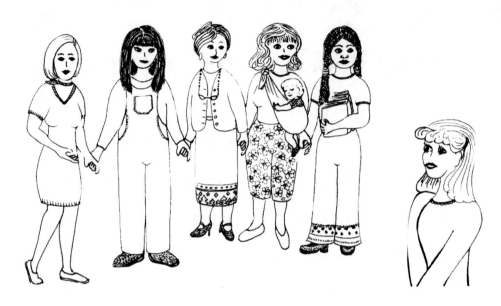

In traditional cultures, a young woman is celebrated as she begins her fertility. She is adorned, honored, instructed, supported, and called upon to begin her journey into her own inner knowing and strength.

No matter what your cultural background, as you begin your moon-time you begin a time of self-discovery, a time of consciously developing your unique talents and gifts. Certainly it is a time to learn what schools and books have to offer, but more importantly it is a time to discover and build your own strengths. *You will find your strengths by following your heart and doing what brings you joy.* Following this very personal inner path will allow you to contribute to life and find fulfillment as a woman. We continue to discover our strengths and talents throughout our lives, but now is when it all begins.

Menopause

Our fertile cycles do not continue forever. Sometime between 40 and 60 years of age, the ovaries stop releasing ova and menstruation no longer occurs. The end of fertility is called menopause and is another phase of the Great Cycle. (2)

Among some indigenous peoples, the post-menopausal women were considered to be dedicated to the well-being of the Earth. The "wise blood," which the older women held within them and did not shed, was considered to give wisdom. It was therefore the domain of the white-haired women to decide what would benefit the planet for seven generations. (5) In the Iroquois Confederation of Native Americans the post-menopausal women named the chiefs. They also attended the clan meetings, standing behind the circle of men who spoke and voted, and removed them from office if they strayed too far from the wishes of the women. (17)

In some traditions, menopause is called the "second spring" because when the childbearing years are over many women discover unexpected energy and creativity. Post-menopausal women often consider this newly found vitality to be a great gift, and use it to pursue long-cherished desires and projects. Before menopause, on the other hand, women often find they reserve a portion of their creativity in case they need it to birth and care for a child. (18)

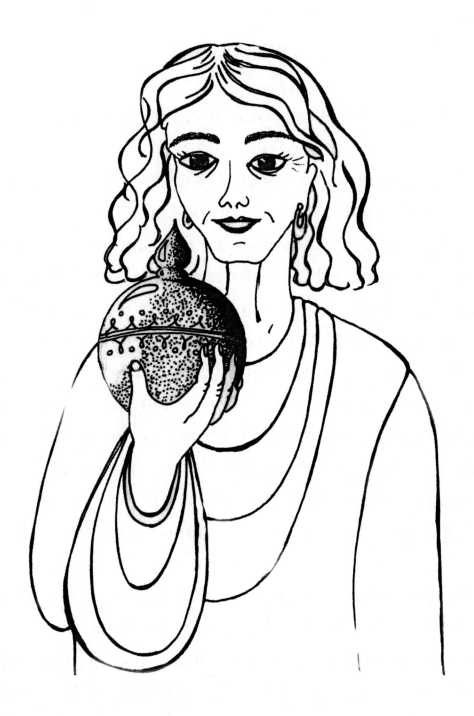

As a "white-haired woman," I extend to you, a young woman beginning the great cycles of Grandmother Moon, my warmest blessings for creativity, inner strength, and fulfillment of your life's purpose. May you enjoy the Full Cycle.

Demeter and Persephone
A Greek Myth

Demeter was the mother of agriculture. Her daughter Persephone helped her to care for the growing crops. When their work was finished, Persephone liked to roam among the wildflowers and pick red poppies.

One day Persephone saw spirits of the dead among the hills. They seemed to her to have lost their direction and were hovering about their old habitats. Persephone asked her mother whether the dead had no one to care for them in their Underworld home.

Demeter admitted she was in charge of caring for the spirits of the dead as well as the growing grain. But she said she had been too busy with the growing crops and birthing animals to visit the dead and care for their needs. Hearing this, Persephone decided to go to the Underworld and carry out this work herself.

Separation from a daughter is always painful for a mother, and Demeter wept as Persephone prepared to leave her. Persephone took red poppies and sheaves of grain to remind her of her life as a young girl. And, although it pained her, Demeter herself showed Persephone the way to the dark chasm that led to the Underworld. And Demeter herself handed Persephone a torch so Persephone could find her way to her chosen work.

Then the Grain Mother kissed her daughter and wept as she disappeared into the dark.

Persephone walked down until she came to an enormous cavern filled with the spirits of the dead. Sitting on a rock, which formed a kind of throne, she called each spirit to her, embraced it, and put a mark of red pomegranate juice on each forehead. Pomegranate juice is considered to be the food of the dead. Persephone's actions represented a kind of initiation, preparing the spirits for their rebirth into the world of the living.

Meanwhile, in the upper world, winter overtook the land. Because Demeter wept for her daughter, all growing plants became dormant and frozen. It was months before Persephone emerged from the Underworld and greeted her mother joyfully. On her daughter's return, Demeter again sent her blessings over the Earth. Crops flourished. Animals gave birth. But part of each year Persephone returns to the Underworld to care for the spirits of the dead. While she is gone, her mother mourns until her return in the spring. (19)

This myth dramatizes every woman's individualization, her journey of separation from her mother. Persephone hears the call to her life's work. Her mother is sorrowful over her separation but knows that her daughter can never find her life's path until she separates herself from her. Therefore, Demeter herself shows her daughter the way to depart. As Persephone leaves, Demeter gives her a light so she can find her way to her life's work. The light also allows Persephone to find her way back home again. The light is her mother's unconditional love and support—the greatest gift of a mother to her daughter. Unconditional love and support is also the greatest gift of all women to each other, for it is the light that will allow each of us to develop into full womanhood.

In the Underworld, Persephone greets each spirit and prepares it for rebirth. Persephone's actions represent facing our emotions, and allowing them to be transformed by self-acceptance and self-love. When Persephone reunites with her mother, she has been enriched by her experience in the Underworld, and consequently the mother-daughter relationship is even more joyful than it previously was. Blessings spread over the entire land. The cycle of separation and return continues, bringing the seasons, variety, and fertility to the entire Earth.

This interpretation is by Rita Kambos and the women of Fairfield, Iowa.

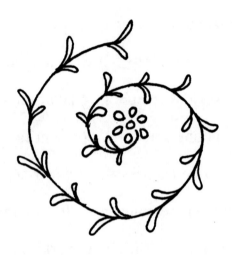

Section Two

Creating the Celebration

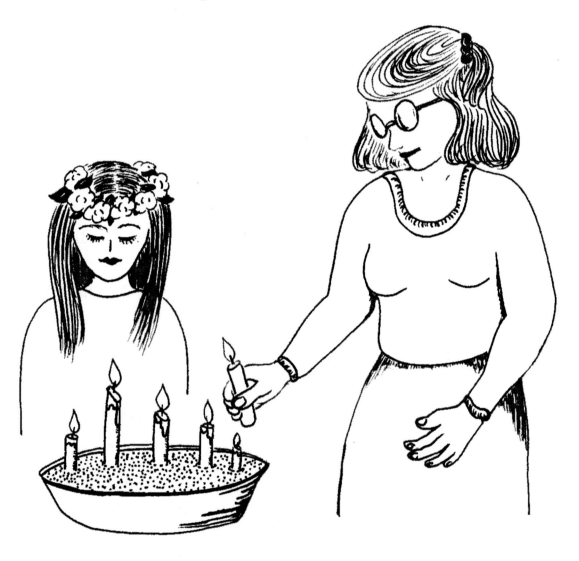

This section is intended for moms as you prepare a ceremony to mark this special time in your daughters' lives. It contains a variety of suggestions for creating rituals that are appropriate for you, your daughters, and your community.

A ritual is usually made up of the following components:

1) Creating and entering a holy space for the ritual. That is, leaving the mundane for the sacred.
2) Invoking the spiritual realm.
3) Building the energy of the ritual.
4) Heart, or high point, of the ritual.
5) Allowing the energy to subside.
6) Closing the ritual.
7) Sharing food and friendship. [1]

The ritual that you create for your daughter should be fun for both of you and for your community of women. So approach this project with a light heart as you choose prayers, songs, and activities that are comfortable for everyone.

Creating a Sacred Space

Choose a comfortable location and create a sacred feeling in whatever way feels comfortable to you and your family. If your ritual is indoors, it is a good idea to turn off the phone ringer and put "Do Not Disturb" signs on the doors. Light candles or incense, play soft music or drum softly, read poetry or sit in silence.

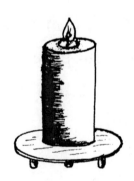

Creating an altar is a common way to create a sacred space. Altars help us remember and focus on what is meaningful for us. The objects on the altar are symbolic of the theme of the ritual. On a first moon-time ritual altar we may have symbols of the Earth, pictures or statues of great or holy women or pictures of women family members. Flowers and other decorations are welcome. A flower crown or garland, which will be worn by the "New Woman," can be on the altar. Another way to create a sacred space is to make a circle with a red rope. Our community of women has a nylon rope, dyed red, which is used at many community rituals.

Dropping the Mundane

This step involves purifying our minds and hearts of daily concerns. It is the intent that is important. You can burn incense, or sprinkle everyone with water, or throw flower petals all around the ritual place—whatever feels to you like purifying the environment.

Smudging is one way to leave behind the cares of daily life. It symbolizes cleaning off negative energy and preparing for the sacred ritual. You can buy smudge sticks at most food co-ops, natural food stores, or stores that sell herbs. Or pick some herbs from your garden, wind cotton string around them to form a "stick" a few inches long and one to three inches in diameter. Hang the herb stick in a warm place and allow it to dry for two to four weeks. At your moon-time ritual, light the stick and "smudge" each other or yourself by letting thc smoke drift around the body.

Ritual seating is another way to separate ourselves from our mundane concerns. In our community of women, we sit in a circle. Young unmarried women sit to the East. Women who have children or are over 25 years of age sit to the South. Women who have passed through menopause sit to the West. And Wise Women sit to the North. Whatever seating you arrange, be sure to reserve a place of honor for the New Woman's grandmother and for grandmother figures.

In most traditions, only women are present at moon-time rituals. The young woman's father, uncles, or brothers, however, are invited to present congratulations and a gift (such as red roses) after the ritual is over. In our community, we do not invite girls who have not yet begun their menstruation to attend a moon-time ritual. This assures that the ritual will be special for them when their time comes. They may join the group when the circle is open for sharing food and friendship.

Invoking the Spiritual Realm

Choosing the prayers for a ritual has to be done carefully. All generations and their beliefs must somehow be honored. This is not always an easy matter. If your tradition contains a concept of the Divine Feminine, now is the time to invoke Her. In our community, we sometimes honor the four directions, which serves as a way to honor nature. In many traditions, nature is considered to be the body of the Divine Feminine.

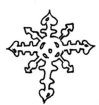

To honor the directions, you can say something like the following:

The East: The East corresponds to the element air, the mind, dawn, spring, pale, airy colors, the eagle and high-flying birds, and the power to know. Young women are keepers of the energy of the East. Their role is to develop their own inner strengths and talents. Welcome to the keepers of the energy of the East.

The South: The South corresponds to the element fire, energy or spirit, noon, summer, fiery reds and oranges, and the quality of will. Artists, musicians, singers, writers, poets, gardeners, cooks, athletes, and especially mothers, are the keepers of the energy of the South. Their role is to create and nurture their families and their own personal creative projects. Welcome to the keepers of the energy of the South.

The West: The West corresponds to the element water, emotions, twilight, autumn, deep purples, sea serpents, dolphins, and the power to dare. From the West comes the courage to face our deepest feelings. Women who have passed through menopause are the keepers of the energy of the West. Their role is to extend their nurturing to the entire planet, and to speak the truth, however hard to face. Welcome to the keepers of the energy of the West.

The North: Because the North Star is the center around which the skies revolve, North is considered the most powerful direction. North corresponds to Planet Earth, the body, midnight, winter, black, and the green of vegetation. From the North comes the power to keep silent, to listen as well as speak, to keep secrets, to know what not to say. Wise Women and Medicine Women are the keepers of the energy of the North. Their role is to instruct and inspire the entire circle of women. Welcome to the keepers of the energy of the North.

Prayer to all directions: The leader may say while smudging or sprinkling water: "Great Spirit, Earth Mother, Guardian Energies of the East, South, West, and North, we ask your blessings on our circle."

Raising the Energy

Raising the energy of the ritual can be done in a variety of ways: women can share their thoughts on womanhood, give blessings to the New Woman, sing, or do anything that appeals to the group. It is good to ask the ritual guests to prepare these things ahead of time. Following are some practices which are often a part of the women's rituals in our community.

New Woman's Footprints

Have ready a dish of clean sand or corn meal. (I use a large clay flower pot base and fill it with sand.) Ask the New Woman to step into the dish of sand or corn meal, leaving her footprints. (Have a towel for the New Woman to wipe her feet afterwards.)

Woman's Blessing

Each woman comes forward, lights a candle, and puts it into the foot prints in the sand or corn meal, which represents the New Woman's journey on Mother Earth. She then gives her woman's blessing, such as: "I am Marie, sister of Georgie Ann, daughter of Selia, granddaughter of Mary Ann and Christina, mother of Christina and Elizabeth, grandmother of Erika, Clara, and Savannah Rose. I ask all the women of my line to bless, teach, and protect (New Woman's name) on her journey through all the cycles of Grandmother Moon."

After each woman has made her blessings, The New Woman lights a candle and puts it into the same dish of sand. She gives her woman's introduction, and accepts the blessings of all the women. "I am………., daughter of………., granddaughter of………., and…….…….. I accept your blessings, and thank you all."

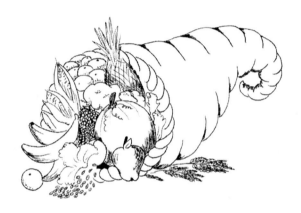

Gifts

If there are gifts for the New Woman, they may be presented now. These gifts may have to do with the New Woman's body and her cycle. If a book is given, it could be about a great woman or somehow have to do with women and women's power or creativity. Jewelry is also traditional. Each gift may be personalized with some words from the person giving the gift. An example is the following: "I am giving you this book because I have always found the life of this great woman to be an inspiration. I know you will find your own creative path and be an equal inspiration to all of us."

Adorning the New Woman

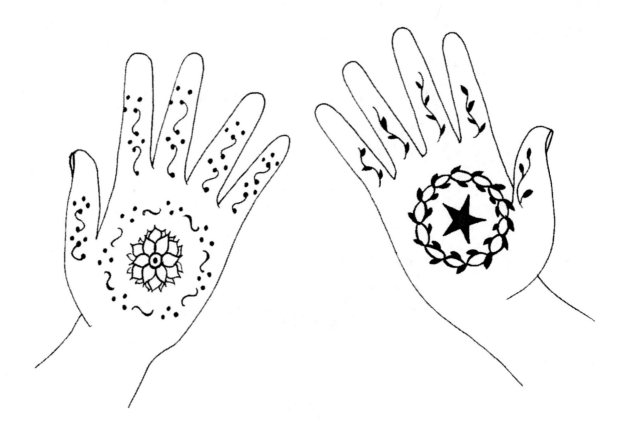

In our community of women, we feel it is important to adorn the New Woman in some way in order to call attention to and honor the changes happening in her body. A flower crown or garland is often used. A crescent moon can be painted in red make-up on the New Woman's forehead. Young girls especially enjoy henna temporary paint on their hands and feet.

Henna is an herb that, when painted on the body, leaves a red/orange stain that turns to brown in 24 hours, and lasts for about two weeks. Henna kits are available with instructions in gift shops, food co-ops, and herb suppliers. Make sure to prepare the henna at least three hours before the start of the ritual. And make sure the ritual guests include someone who is artistic or at least courageous enough to do the henna painting.

Some groups of women paint henna lines down the inside of the New Woman's leg. This practice is taken from the Hopi Dance of the Maidens and calls direct attention to the young woman's menstrual flow. If henna is not compatible with your life-style, honor the New Woman with flowers, new clothing, or whatever feels right to your community.

In some cultural groups, the New Woman's hair is put into a bun for the first time in her life and covered by a small white cap. The bun distinguishes the women from the girls, who are still wearing their hair in braids. Gifts in these communities are often associated with the traditional women's work of the community, or may be homemaking items that can be saved by the New Woman for her own home. Create your own way to honor your daughter as she enters womanhood.

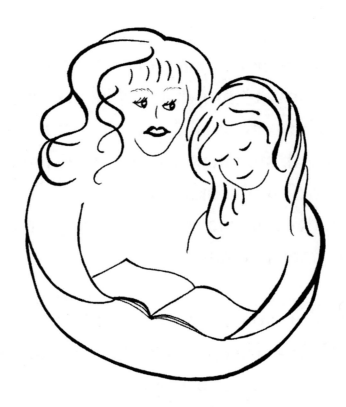

Poems and Stories

It's inspiring at a woman's ritual to hear poems or stories about women from your own community. Ask your friends and family members. You may find some unexpected poets or storytellers.

Mythology

Myths teach eternal truths through imaginary stories. They are time-honored teaching tools that you may enjoy incorporating into your ritual. Throughout this book I have included myths from around the world that teach important truths for young women. See the book list at the back of this book for more sources for mythology.

A Legend of the Knights of the Round Table

King Arthur had accepted a quest to discover, in less than one year and under the pain of death, what a woman wants above all else. The year was drawing to a close and King Arthur had not been able to fulfill his quest. He considered asking the help of a famous, but ugly, witch who was reputed to have great wisdom. He hesitated, however, because the witch demanded a high price for any help she gave. Finally, left with no other choice, King Arthur visited the witch with his question.

"Above all else," the witch replied, "a woman desires sovereignty over herself. And for my payment I will take your finest knight to be my husband."

Now King Arthur went to Sir Gawain and said, "Here is your fair lady. You will be her knight protector."

Sir Gawain was an honorable man. He treated the witch with utmost respect and honor during their engagement period. On their wedding night, the ugly witch appeared to Sir Gawain in radiant beauty—a goddess beyond any earthly woman.

The witch, now a beautiful goddess, said to Sir Gawain, "I can be as you see me now, all day every day, or all night every night. Which do you choose?"

Sir Gawain thought in silence for some time before he replied, "My lady, you must choose." With these words the witch became beautiful both by day and by night. (20)

King Arthur represents physical existence. Sir Gawain represents the mind. The witch/goddess represents intuition, or heart. Physical means alone are unable to accomplish the goal, and King Arthur asks the help of the witch, the heartfelt knowing. The heart demands marriage with Sir Gawain, the mind.

In this way, an inner harmony is achieved. The physical senses encounter life's challenges. The mind thinks and reasons, but allows the intuitive knowing to give direction. With the harmonious marriage of body, mind and heart, we gain sovereignty over ourselves and walk in beauty both by day and by night.

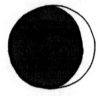

Shiva and Parvati
A Story from Ancient India

A demon once did great spiritual exercises and gained enough power to bring the entire universe under his control. The only being who would be able to break the spell was the son of Shiva. Shiva, the god of destruction and transformation, was a renunciate, however, and never left his meditation. He had no son and no interest in fathering a child, for renunciates only desire spiritual union with Universal Consciousness.

From heaven the gods made a plan to save the world from the spell of the demon. They sent Parvati, the most beautiful of goddesses, to call Shiva from his meditation and produce a divine son who could save the world. Parvati tried in every way to interest Shiva in love. She painted her eyes and lips. She put bells on her ankles and danced the sacred dances. She played the vena, a sacred stringed instrument, and sang the sacred songs of nature. Nothing took Shiva's attention away from his meditation. Finally the gods sent Kama, the god of lust, to shoot Shiva with one of his powerful flower arrows that cause their victims to be filled with sexual desire.

Opening his third eye, Shiva burned Kama to ashes with a glance, without so much as leaving his meditation.

Unable to interest Shiva in love, and unable to return to the gods without giving birth to Shiva's son, Parvati was filled with disappointment with the world. She became determined to seek Self-realization. She walked to the mountains, sat down on the ground, and began to meditate. Parvati sat in silence for many months, her mind fixed on the Divine.

It was then that Shiva, deep within his meditation, began to feel an energy, a powerful awareness, as vast as his own. Opening his three eyes, he saw Parvati seated in meditation in ecstatic union with the Divine. The gods smiled from heaven. They realized Shiva had fallen in love, and they foresaw the birth of the world's savior.

By seeking the highest within herself, Parvati saved the world. In the same way, every woman, by following her highest inner knowing, brings love and blessings to her world. (21)

Mother's Prayer

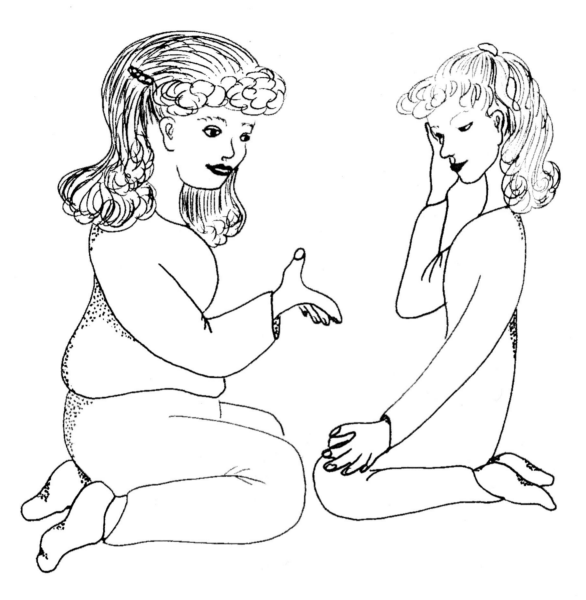

This is an important part of building the spiritual energy of the ritual: the New Woman's mother prays for her daughter. She can compose her own prayer or choose a prayer that is comfortable for her. Mother and daughter can kneel or sit facing each other during this prayer. In our community we sometimes use the following Native American prayer:

Native American Mother's Prayer

Ho, green things, trees, flowers, grasses.
Hear my voice.
Listen, come bless us. Hear me.
Make space for this New Woman,
that she may walk the brow of the first hill.

Ho, rocks, things of the ground, Ancient Ones,
hear my voice. I'm on my knees to you.
Make space for this good daughter.
Help her,
that she may walk the brow of the second hill.

Ho, things of the air, winged ones,
hear my voice. I'm calling to you.
Make space for this new wise one.
Please, I'm on my knees to you.
Consent, that she may walk the brow of the third hill.

Ho, four legged ones, all the animals,
things that creep and crawl, hear my voice.
I'm calling to you.
I'm asking you on my hands and knees
that you make space for this New Woman.
Help her,
that she may walk the brow of the fourth hill.

Ho, green things that grow, things that fly in the air,
things that walk on the Earth,
Four-legged ones, hear my voice.
Make space for this good woman.
Help her to walk singing over the brow of many hills.

(Everyone says: Ho!)

Daughter's Prayer

The New Woman now makes her own prayer. She may recite a prayer or poem of her choosing or one she has composed herself. Following is "The Daughter's Prayer," taken from the Navajo Puberty Ritual.

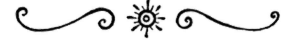

Navajo Daughter's Prayer

Hold your hand before me in protection.
Stand guard for me. Speak in defense of me.
Do what I ask of you.
I will do what you ask of me.
May it be beautiful before me.
May it be beautiful behind me.
May it be beautiful below me.
May it be beautiful above me.
May it be beautiful around me.
I am restored in beauty.
I am restored in beauty.
I am restored in beauty.
I am restored in beauty.

Heart of the Ritual

The central point of any ritual usually involves some symbolic passage. In a marriage it is the vows. In a graduation it is the distribution of diplomas. In a baby shower it may be the opening of gifts for the baby. In a first moon-time ritual the high point usually involves the New Woman's acceptance of her role as a woman. Women have invented a variety of ways to create a passage for their daughters. As one example, the women at the ritual stand in two lines with arms raised, forming an archway. The New Woman stands at the entrance to the archway. She holds a few toys representing her childhood. She has been asked to bring the toys to the ritual to be given to the younger children of the community. However, she is not asked to bring all her toys, or her favorite toy, because aspects of the child remain within all of us and continue to be treasured throughout our lives.

The young woman's grandmother leads the passage ritual. If her grandmother is not present, then a grandmother figure may be chosen to represent her. Wise Woman asks, "Who approaches this passage?" New Woman gives her name. Wise Woman continues, "When you are ready to leave behind your childhood and become a member of the circle of women, leave your toys behind, and walk through the arch." New Woman puts down her toys and walks through the arch. As she comes to the end of the arch, the women ring bells, throw flower petals, and cheer. Everyone kisses and hugs the New Woman.

Allowing the Energy of the Ritual to Subside

Now that the high point of the ritual is over, it is an easy matter to allow the energy to settle again.

Singing together is one way to allow the energy to settle gently, while maintaining the sacred atmosphere. You may enjoy some of the songs on the CD called "Songs for the Inner Child" by Shaina Noll. Following are some other songs that we have used at our community's moon-time rituals. You can sing any one as a round.

Woman Am I

Anonymous

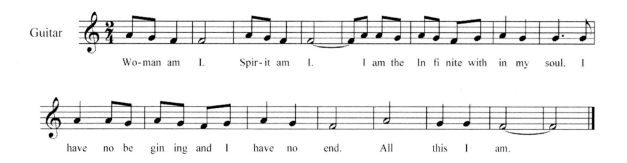

Love

Anonymous

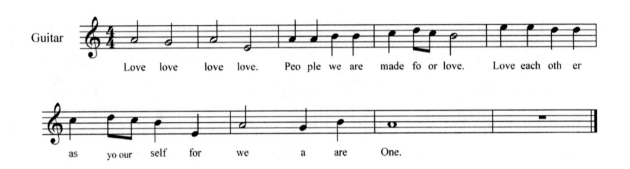

Love love love love. Peo ple we are made fo or love. Love each oth er

as yo our self for we a are One.

River of Life

Anonymous

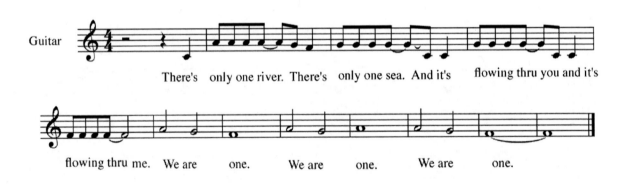

There's only one river. There's only one sea. And it's flowing thru you and it's

flowing thru me. We are one. We are one. We are one.

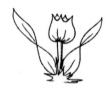

Grandmother Moon

Marie Zenack

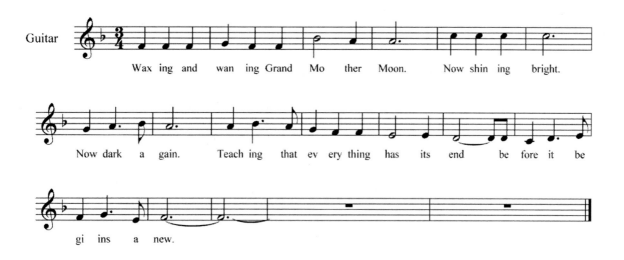

Closing the Ritual

The sacred space is now opened to the more mundane activities of eating and drinking. In the rituals of our community we usually say a closing prayer and wind up the red rope. The closing prayer marks the end of the ritual. No one likes to drag a ritual on too long after the heart of the ritual is over, so keep the closing prayer short. Choose something compatible with your beliefs and comfortable for your community. Two possible prayers follow.

Native American Prayer for Peace

May peace prevail on Earth.

May peace prevail in my mind.

May peace prevail in my heart.

May peace prevail in my life.

May I know peace.

May my ancestors know peace.

May my children's children know peace unto seven generations.

May peace prevail on Earth.

Traditional Prayer to Mother Earth

By the Earth that is Her body,

By the air that is Her breath,

By the fire that is Her bright spirit,

By the living waters of Her womb,

The circle is open, but unbroken.

The peace of the Goddess go in our hearts.

Merry meet, merry part, and merry meet again. Blessed be.

Share Food and Friendship

The men of the family, and the young girls who have not yet begun their moon-time, can now be invited to congratulate the New Women and join in the eating and friendship. (22)

Section Three

Sexuality and Birth

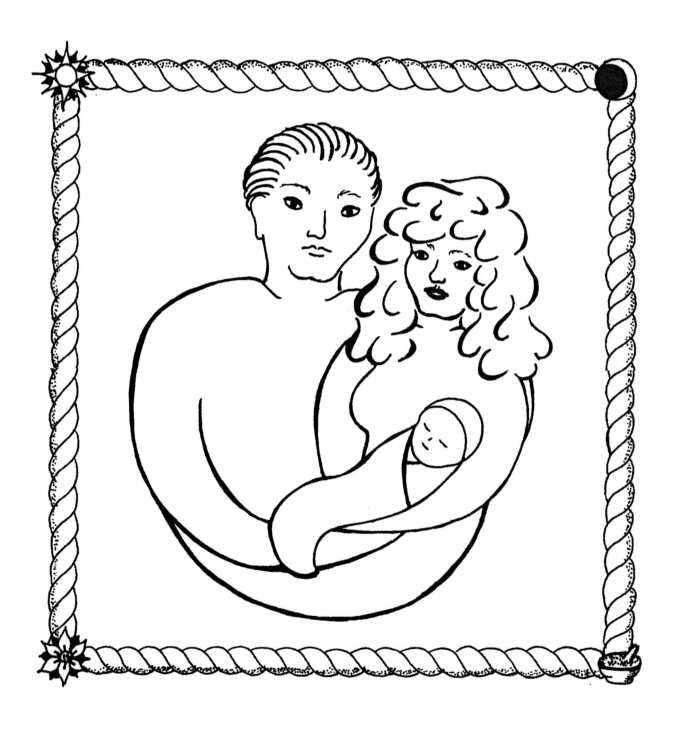

More About the Woman's Reproductive Cycle

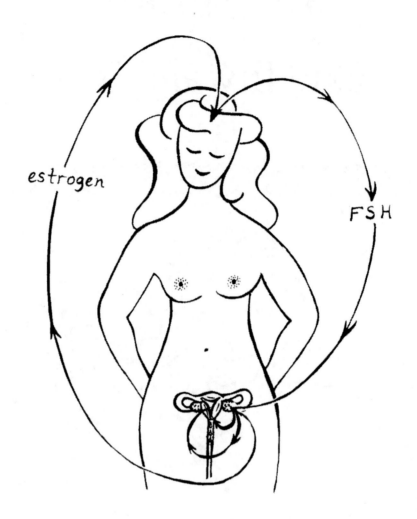

Let's take a look at the cycle of fertility in more detail. To begin the cycle, a hormone, called follicle-stimulating hormone, (FSH) is produced by the pituitary gland in the brain. FSH travels through the bloodstream to the ovaries, causing a few of the many tiny follicles there to begin ripening, or maturing. Each follicle is a tiny ring of cells with a tiny ovum, or egg, inside. As the follicles ripen, they produce another hormone, called estrogen. Estrogen causes the cervix, the opening of the uterus, to begin making moisture and mucus. This is when we notice wetness or mucus outside the vagina.

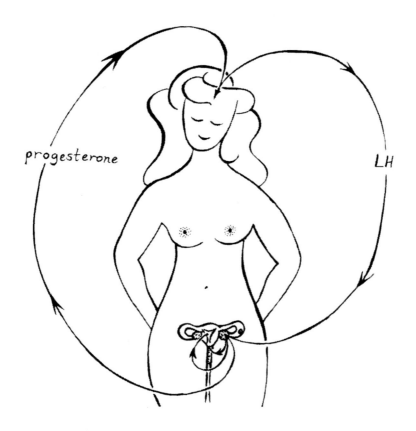

Estrogen also causes the endometrium, the lining of the uterus, to grow soft and spongy, forming a kind of bed that can hold and nourish a baby. Finally, estrogen signals the pituitary gland in the brain that some follicles have matured in the ovaries.

When the pituitary gland receives the message that some follicles have matured, it produces another hormone, leutenizing hormone, or LH. LH causes one of the ripening follicles to release its ovum into a fallopian tube. The ovum travels along the fallopian tube for 12 to 24 hours. If pregnancy does not occur during that time, it disintegrates and is reabsorbed by the body.

The empty follicle, which is called the corpus luteum, lives for about another two weeks, all the while making progesterone, another hormone. Progesterone thickens the fertile-type mucus in the cervix, creating a plug to keep infection out of the uterus in case of a pregnancy. Progesterone also causes the endometrium to continue growing soft and spongy. And finally, progesterone stops the pituitary in the brain from sending any more hormonal messages to begin another cycle. Progesterone continues to delay the beginning of another cycle for about two weeks, when the empty follicle dies. (23) (By the way, you don't have to memorize this. Your body will work just right anyway.)

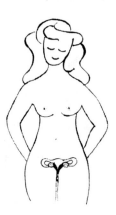

When the empty follicle dies and pregnancy has not occurred, the lining of the uterus is shed with menstruation. The bloody menstrual flow is actually the lining of the uterus that would have held and nourished a baby if this had been the time in our lives to become moms.

More about Hormones and Emotions

During the days when the ova are ripening in our ovaries and the fertile mucus is present in our vaginas, we may feel courageous and loving. Young men who bored us last week may suddenly appear interesting and attractive. These emotions and reactions are caused by the hormone estrogen, which is getting us ready to have a baby, even though we may not want that for ourselves yet!

These hormonal urges have to be safely navigated by all women throughout our years of fertility. Charting our cycle, with its signs and signals, helps to keep us aware of the waxing and waning of emotions and sexual desire. This awareness, called fertility awareness, allows us to harness the energies of our cycle to power our own life goals, rather than allowing our hormones to push us in ways we really do not want to go.

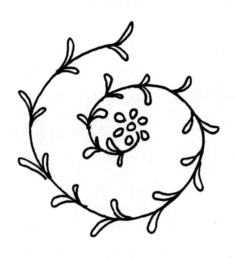

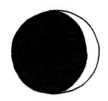

Charting Your Moon-time Cycle

Look at the three moon-time charts on the next page. The woman has marked the days of menstruation with the word "red." She has left the days blank when she felt nothing and saw nothing outside the vagina. The woman drew raindrops on the chart when she felt or saw *something*—moisture, creaminess, mucus—outside the vaginal opening. *Something* may be only pasty or creamy mucus, or a wet feeling, but it indicates possible fertility. She colored the raindrops dark on days when she felt a *slippery* wetness. The last day of *any* slippery, wet feeling is the probable day of ovulation, the release of the ovum from the ovaries, and the day of maximum fertility. Fertility continues for the following three or four days. Infertile days cannot be known for certain without additional information. Please see Endnote 24.

As these charts demonstrate, cycles vary in length. Bleeding may last three to five days, or even longer. Wet days can vary in number. The length of the dry time before the wet time begins can also vary. Each cycle is unique and each woman is unique. But when the slippery wetness returns to sticky or dry, you can count ahead about two weeks to predict your time of bleeding. You will soon learn your unique time.

May 2005

Sun	Mon	Tue	Wed	Thu	Fri	Sat
1 Red	2 Red	3 Red	4 Spots	5	6	7
8	9	10	11	12 ⬭	13 ⬭	14 ⬤
15 ⬤⬤	16 ⬤⬤⬤	17 ⬤⬤⬤	18	19	20	21
22	23	24	25	26	27	28
29	30	31 Red				

June 2005

Sun	Mon	Tue	Wed	Thu	Fri	Sat
			1 Red	2 Red	3 Red	4 Spots
5	6	7	8	9	10 ⬭	11 ⬤
12 ⬤⬤	13 ⬤⬤⬤	14 ⬤	15	16	17	18
19	20	21	22	23	24	25
26	27	28 Red	29 Red	30 Red		

July 2005

Sun	Mon	Tue	Wed	Thu	Fri	Sat
					1 Spots	2
3	4	5	6	7	8	9
10	11	12 ⬭	13 ⬤	14 ⬤⬤	15 ⬤⬤⬤	16 ⬤
17	18	19	20	21	22	23
24	25	26	27	28	29	30
31 Red						

To be sure of your exact fertile time, it is necessary to learn, from a fertility awareness teacher or book, how to observe and chart other signs of fertility, such as resting body temperature and position of the cervix. (24) But charting your cervical mucus will put you in tune with your feelings and allow you to predict your days of bleeding with accuracy.

The Male Hormonal System

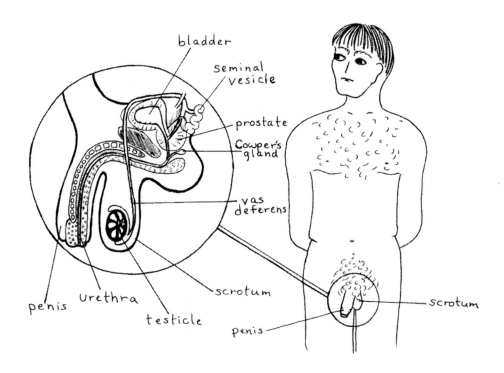

Young men's bodies also go through changes in preparation for becoming fathers. The pituitary gland in the brain sends a hormone, called follicle-stimulating hormone, (FSH) to the testicles, which are the male sex glands. FSH signals the testicles to produce sperm, which are the male reproductive cells.

Sperm are so small they can only be seen through a microscope. Each tiny sperm has a tail that allows it to move. After sperm are produced in the testicles, they travel through a tube called the vas deferens to the seminal vesicle, which holds the mature sperm.

A gland called the prostate makes seminal fluid, which is the fluid that will transport the sperm in the urethra. The urethra is a tube extending from the bladder, through the prostate, and through the penis to the outside of the man's body.

During sexual activity, the prostate gland becomes as full of fluid as it can comfortably hold, and it contracts (squeezes). As the prostate contracts, it draws sperm from the seminal vesicle. Seminal fluid mixed with sperm is called semen. The contractions of the prostate gland force the semen through the urethra and out the tip of the penis.(25) This is called ejaculation. The ejaculate (semen) is a teaspoon to a tablespoon of thick milky liquid and contains millions of microscopic sperm.

During sexual activity, but before ejaculation, the penis becomes engorged with blood. This causes the penis to become firm and erect, and is called the male erection. The male erection allows the penis to pass into the vagina of the woman.

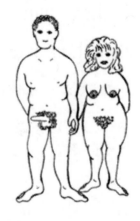

Once ejaculation has deposited the sperm in the woman's vagina, they swim up the vagina to the uterus. They swim in the cervical mucus that is produced during the fertile, wet time of our cycle. The secretions of the vagina are normally acidic to protect us from infections. The cervical mucus, produced during our fertile, wet time, is alkaline and protects the sperm from the acidic environment of the vagina. It also filters out imperfect sperm and guides the healthy sperm up into the uterus. From there, the sperm swim into the fallopian tubes.

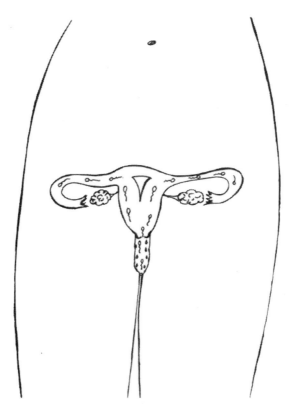

(In the illustration, the microscopic sperm have been drawn much bigger than their actual size.) They do not know which fallopian tube may contain the ovum, and so they swim both ways!

Urination and Ejaculation

Even though the urethra transports both urine and semen through the penis to the outside of the man's body, when a man has an erection a valve closes between the prostate gland and the bladder to prevent urine from being released when semen is ejaculated. Practically speaking, this means that a man cannot urinate and ejaculate at the same time. (26)

As women, we know that, even though our bodies may be making cervical mucus, we are not necessarily ready to be moms. Similarly, young men begin having erections long before they are ready to be dads. This is all a natural part of growing up.

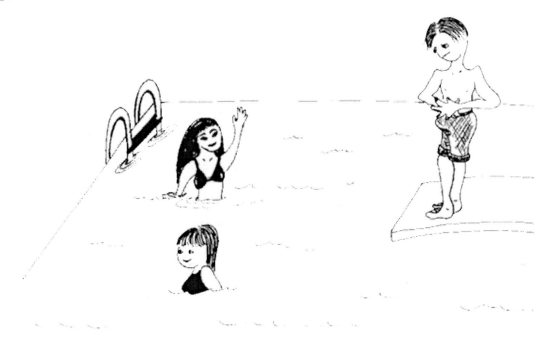

The male hormone involved in the production of sperm is testosterone. Testosterone can cause a young man to feel competitive, aggressive, and very interested in women. However, successful men everywhere have learned to harness their hormonal energy to fulfill their life goals, rather than allowing their hormones to direct their lives.

Feeding the Wolves

A Native American grandfather was talking to his young grandson.

"I have two wolves inside of me," he told the boy, "and they are struggling with each other. The first is the wolf of peace, love, and kindness. The other is the wolf of fear, greed, and hatred."

"Which wolf will win, grandfather?" asked the young boy.

"Whichever one I feed," replied the grandfather.

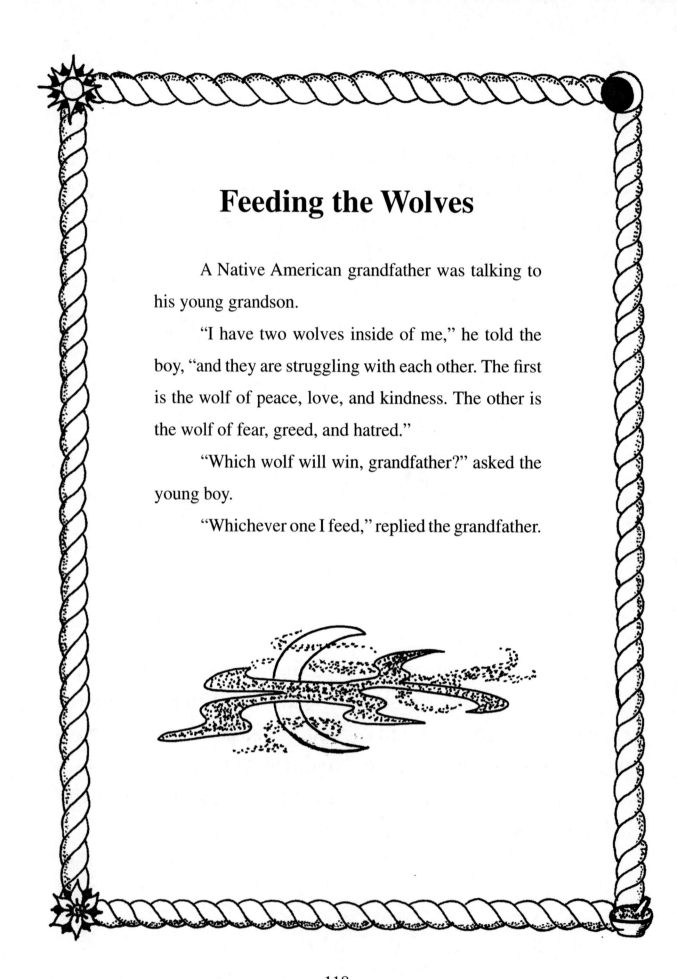

Making Love

The sexual union between a man and a woman is called sexual intercourse. However, nobody really calls it that. We call it making love because, when a man and a woman build a life together, sexual intercourse is part of what brings love, joy, forgiveness and commitment to their union. Usually couples make love in bed because it is comfortable and private.

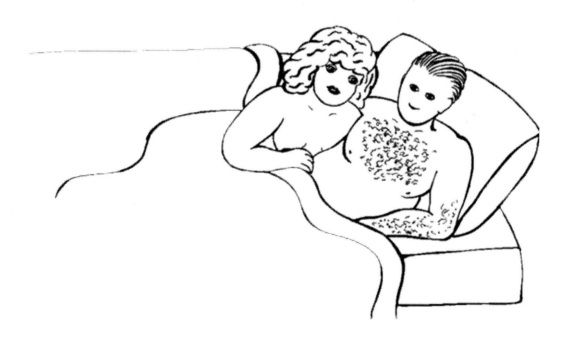

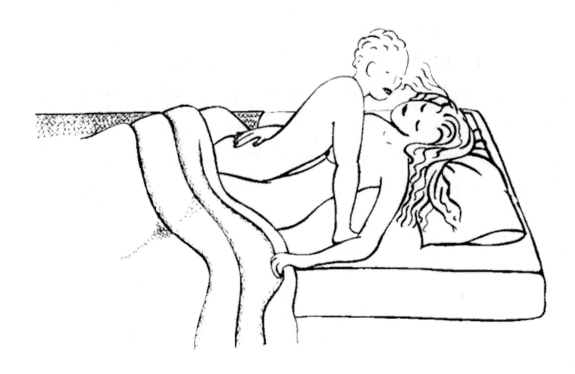

Feeling loved and cared for is important for the enjoyment of making love.

Engagement and Marriage

In many traditional cultures, the engagement period lasts one full year, and is considered to be a time of preparation for marriage. During the engagement the couple gets to know each other's temperament, which is thought to vary with the change of seasons.

Most cultures agree that having sexual relations creates a bond that is difficult to break without heartache. For this reason the traditional engagement period is a time of friendship without sexual relations. The year of engagement allows the couple to know if they feel deep ease, respect, and happiness in each other's company, before making a life commitment.

Couples who begin sexual relations early in their friendship may find themselves unhappily staying together only to avoid the pain of separation. They also risk unintended pregnancy and sexually transmitted diseases (STDs), which are diseases passed from one person to another through intimate contact. See the end notes for sources of information on sexually transmitted diseases.
(28)

Conception

On the opposite page is a close-up view of conception, which is the beginning of pregnancy. The couple has made love, and the sperm have travelled from the woman's vagina, through her uterus, and into the fallopian tube to meet the ovum.

When a sperm penetrates the ovum, it is called fertilization. Even without ejaculation, sperm are present in the small amount of fluid produced by a tiny gland called the Cowper's gland. Cowper's fluid leaks out of the penis during sexual activity. Therefore pregnancy is possible even without ejaculation.

Even without penetration of the man's penis inside the woman's vagina, when there is fertile-type mucus in the woman's body, the tiny, microscopic sperm can swim into the vaginal opening, up the vagina, into the uterus, and into the fallopian tubes. There the sperm may meet the ovum, and pregnancy may begin.

For this reason, during the woman's fertile time, pregnancy is possible with only genital contact (touching of the penis to the vaginal area). (6)

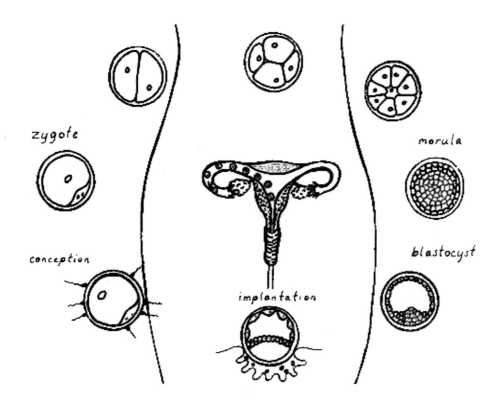

zygote

morula

conception

blastocyst

implantation

Dividing and maturing as it goes, the fertilized ovum is moved slowly along the fallopian tube toward the uterus by the cilia, tiny hairs inside the fallopian tubes. In six or seven days, the fertilized ovum implants in the endometrium (the lining of the uterus), the bed that has been created to receive it. Menstruation (bleeding) does not occur, because the fertilized ovum, growing and developing in the uterus, creates hormones that maintain the uterine lining. The woman realizes she has conceived. (6)

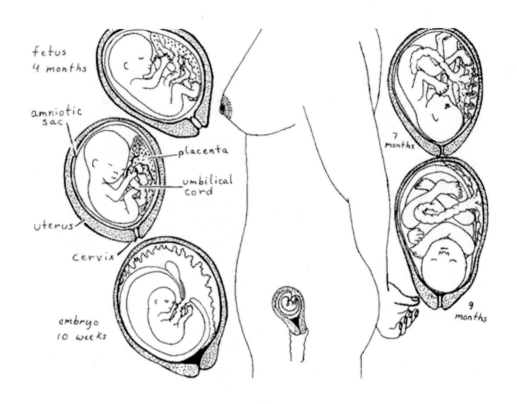

fetus
4 months

amniotic
sac

placenta

umbilical
cord

uterus

cervix

embryo
10 weeks

7
months

9
months

Pregnancy

You are already caring for your baby today, even though motherhood is a long way off for you. The ovum that someday may be fertilized to form the body of your child is present even now in your body. Eating well and avoiding taking unhealthy substances into your body today is the beginning of caring for your baby tomorrow.

During pregnancy, nutrition and healthy habits become even more important. Moms who eat well and exercise sensibly will enjoy their pregnancies more.

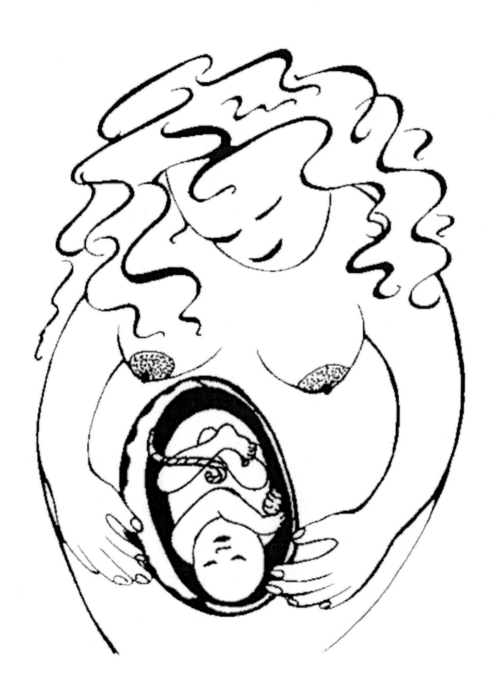

Labor

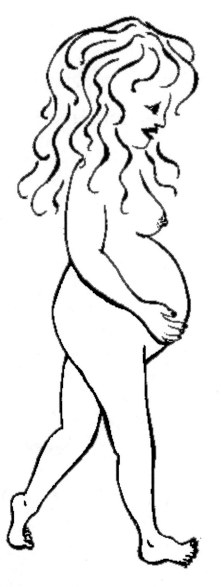

The hormonal changes that happen during labor and birth prepare the mother to nurture her child during the many years ahead. (29) Birthing is probably the single most difficult yet most fulfilling thing a woman will do in her life. It is no wonder, when a woman is giving birth, we say she is "in labor." Sometimes a woman feels "I cannot do it."

This is when the support of other women who have already given birth becomes important. For the laboring mom, remaining active and trying different positions, especially leaning forward, can ease the discomfort. (30)

Some women choose to give birth with a midwife, at home or in birthing centers that allow them to choose the birth experience they desire.

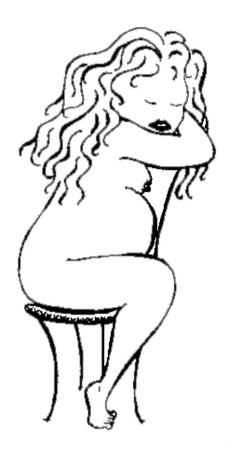

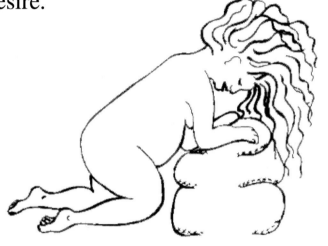

Birth

Even though our vaginas may seem small, they contain folds and are elastic. When a woman is giving birth, the vagina unfolds and stretches to allow the baby to be born. Giving birth is a rite of passage for women—a life-changing effort that can take us to a new level of womanly expression. Many women say the power they felt while laboring and birthing empowered their entire creative life.

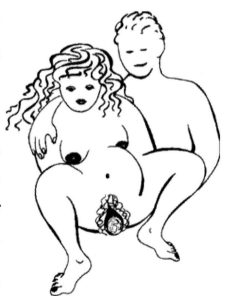

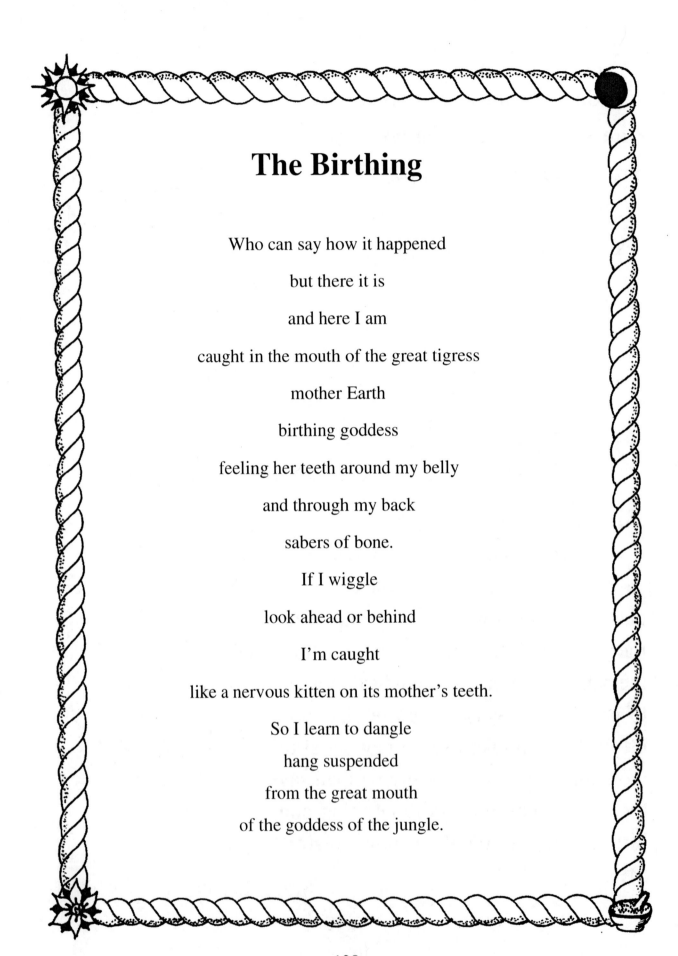

The Birthing

Who can say how it happened

but there it is

and here I am

caught in the mouth of the great tigress

mother Earth

birthing goddess

feeling her teeth around my belly

and through my back

sabers of bone.

If I wiggle

look ahead or behind

I'm caught

like a nervous kitten on its mother's teeth.

So I learn to dangle

hang suspended

from the great mouth

of the goddess of the jungle.

Surrender.

Until her movement is mine

and I am pacing

turning

bending

still loose—

suspended.

And I roar.

Feeling her pass through me

great mother

my lover

as we are born

and lie together.

Tiny child.

My body curled around

like a tigress and her cub.

-By Christina Wadsworth

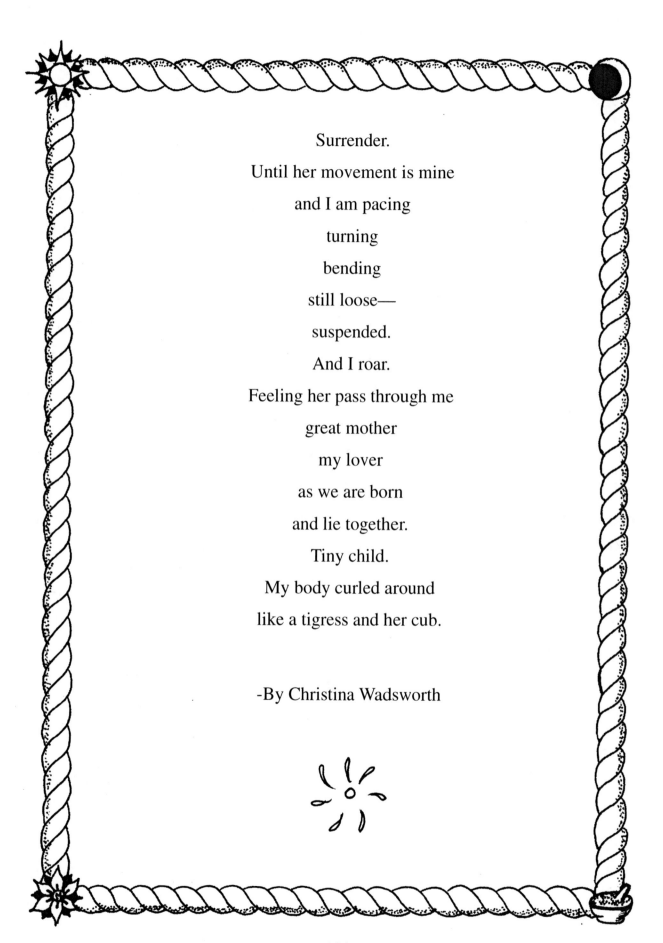

Breastfeeding

A mother's breasts produce milk for her baby. Breast milk contains the perfect nutrition for baby. It also contains the mother's immunities to disease, which protect baby in the early months of life. Equally important, breast milk comes with all the love and closeness of mother. It is no accident babies are born knowing how to suck from their mother's breasts, and it is no wonder breasts are considered beautiful in all cultures.

A mother's breasts begin to produce milk two or three days after the birth of her baby. Before the milk "comes in," the breasts produce colostrum, a pre-milk liquid that cleanses and prepares baby's digestion. Frequent breastfeedings during the first few days after the birth serve to bond mother and baby, build baby's immunity to disease, and bring in mother's milk more smoothly.

The hormone involved in milk production, called oxytocin, makes breastfeeding pleasurable for the mother and causes her to feel tenderness and love for her baby. Oxytocin also causes a mother's uterus to quickly shrink back to its pre-pregnancy size. (31)

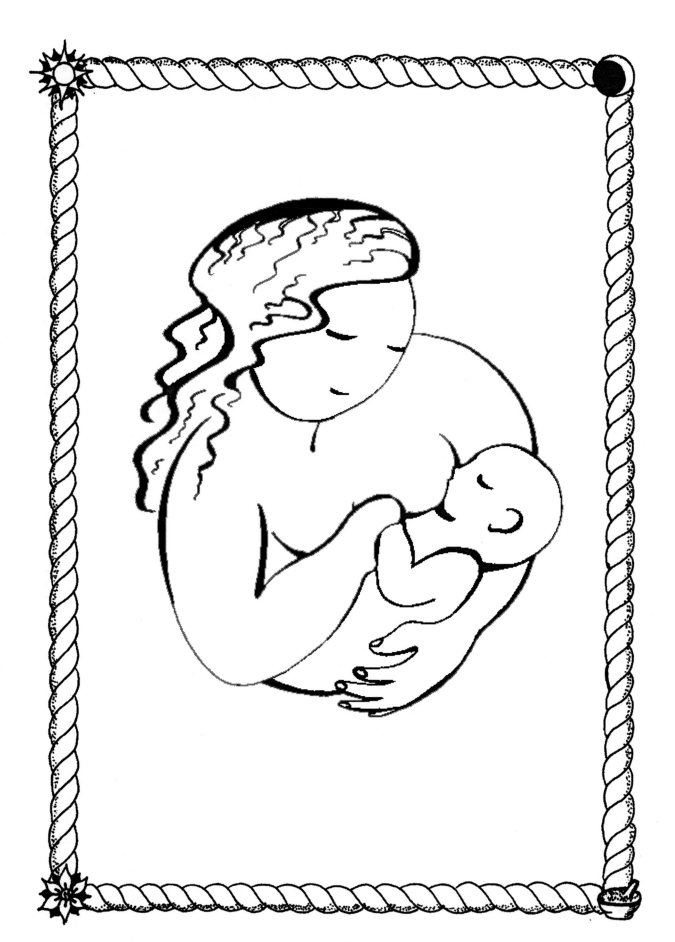

Love and Our Breasts

Feelings of tenderness and love, the result of the hormone oxytocin, are also produced during sexual activity. When the breasts are caressed or stimulated, tender feelings arise that cause a woman to bond (feel united) with her sexual partner. This bonding occurs even if her sexual partner does not return her affection. The "love" she feels is the result of oxytocin. (29)

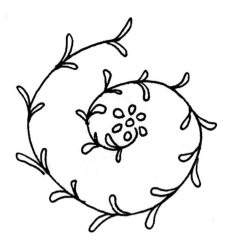

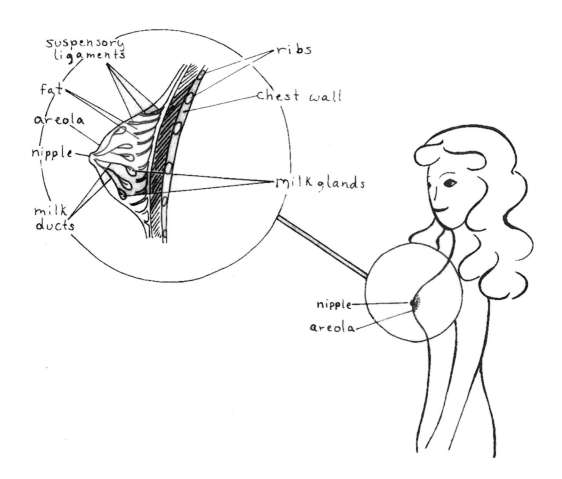

Each of our breasts contains fifteen to twenty alveoli, or milk glands. Each alveoli is drained by a duct opening on the surface of the nipple. The alveoli are surrounded by fatty and fibrous tissue, making our breasts soft. Ligaments at the top of the breasts suspend them, and give them shape. In the breasts of nursing moms, droplets of milk pass through the small ducts and are stored in reservoirs just behind the nipple. The baby's sucking causes more milk to let down from the alveoli toward the nipple. (31)

Motherhood

Motherhood is a great gift, bringing a special kind of fulfillment to a woman's creative energies. It is also a lifelong job, requiring constant sacrifice and attention. Motherhood is not for all women. We are all, however, meant to develop our unique creative and nurturing energies and contribute our own special gifts to Mother Earth.

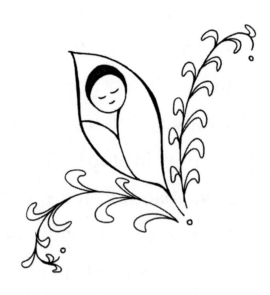

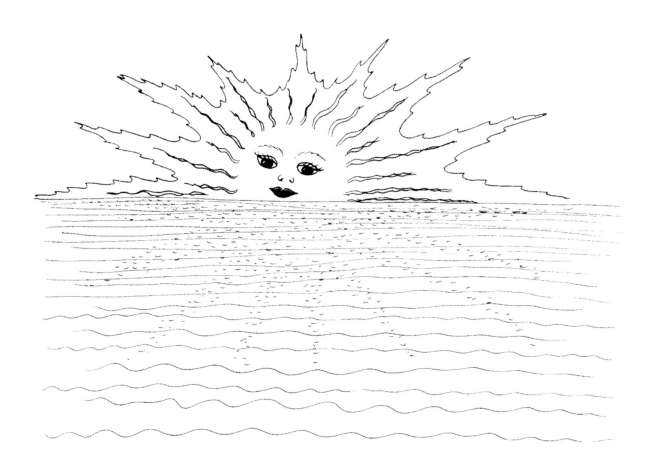

May we all find our gifts and let them shine.

White Buffalo Calf Woman
A Native American Legend

The story of White Buffalo Calf Woman dates back to a time, centuries ago, when the people of the Lakota Native American tribe were living out of harmony with nature. As a result of the lack of harmony with Nature, the rains did not come on time, there were no buffalo, and the people were starving.

The tribe sent two young warriors out across the plains to look for buffalo. As their eyes scanned the distance, the young men saw a woman walking across the prairie. As she approached, they saw she was beautiful. One of the young men, seeing that the woman was alone and without the protection of her people, approached her to take advantage of her. As he drew near to her, a cloud encircled them both. When it cleared, there was nothing left of the young warrior but a pile of bones at White Buffalo Calf Woman's feet.

The other young man was a true warrior and knew when you find something beautiful, it is not for yourself but for your people. So he said, "Strange and beautiful woman, may I take you to my people?" She replied, "Yes. Go before me, and build a lodge for me."

So it happened that White Buffalo Calf Woman lived among the Lakota people for many years, giving them the ceremonial peace pipe and all the ceremonies they needed to restore harmony with Nature.

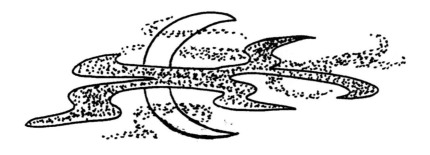

Legends and myths are more than stories that happened a long time ago: they are stories that happen in all of our lives. Every woman is approached by two different kinds of men, two different kinds of warriors. The first seeks to take advantage of us for his own purposes. But the true warrior knows we do not belong to him. We belong to ourselves and to our people. So he says, "May I take you to my people?" and "Teach us to live in harmony with the cycles of nature." (5)

Recommended Reading

Women Who Run With the Wolves, by Clarissa Pinkola Estés

The most powerful of storytellers, Clarissa recounts myths from around the globe and analyses these myths in the light of women's spiritual evolution. Try reading only one story at a time, giving it time to work its magic before reading another.

Nourishing Traditions, by Sally Fallon

The author has really done her homework in this cookbook that is also a life changing nutrition course. Her health information and recipes are based on extensive scientific study of health producing traditional eating, rather than on fads or commercial food interests. Delicious meals that transformed my family's health.

The Thundering Years, by Julie Tallard Johnson

Recommended for both young people and their parents, this book gives an understanding of the strong energies of the young, as well as ways to honor and channel those energies through mentoring and ritual.

Herbal Healing for Women, by Rosemary Gladstar

The author describes how to prepare natural herbal treatments for the healing and comfort of women of all ages.

Everybody's Guide to Homeopathic Medicines, by Stephen Cummings, M.D., and Dana Ullman, M.P.H.

Learn to care for yourself and your family with safe, inexpensive, and effective remedies.

Hormone Heresy, and *Protect Your Daughter from Breast Cancer,*

both by Sherrill Sellman.

These books give candid information about the dangers of artificial hormones for women of all ages.

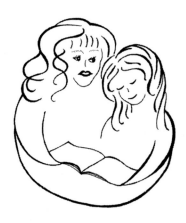

End Notes

1. Johnson, Julie Tallard. *The Thundering Years: Rituals and Sacred Wisdom for Teens.* Rochester, Vermont: Bindu Books, 2001, pp.93-138.

2. Billings, Evelyn. *The Billings Method, Every Woman's Guide to Her Reproductive System.* New York: Ballantine Books, a division of Random House, Inc., 1980, pp. 68-119.

3. Federation of Feminist Women's Centers. *A New View of a Woman's Body.* West Hollywood, CA: 1991, p. 70.

4. Singer, Sydney and Soma Grismaijer. *Dressed to kill.* Garden City Park, New York: Avery Publishing Group, 1995, pp. 99-121.

5. Medicine Eagle, Brooke. Moon Time, audio recording. Singing Eagle Enterprises, PMB C 401, Polson, MT. http://www.MedicineEagle.com.

6. Wilson, Mercedes, *Love and Fertility.* Dunkirk, MD: Family of the Americas Foundation, 1998, pp. 28-51.

7. Sjoo, Monica and Barbara Mor. *The Great Cosmic Mother: Rediscovering the Religion of the Earth.* San Francisco: Harper, 1991, pp. 144-149.

8. United States National Toxicology Program, <u>Report on Carcinogens</u>, Tenth Edition. http://ntp-server.niehs.nih.gov/

9. United States Food and Drug Administration. <u>On the Teen Scene, Good News About Good Nutrition</u>: FDA Consumer, April, 1992. http://www.cfsan.fda.gov/

10. Richardson, Terra. <u>Ayurveda and Menses for Wisewomen</u>. http://www. wisewomanhood.com/womenshealthmenstrualhealth.htm.

11. Witmer, Denise. <u>Parenting of Adolescents: Teenagers and Sleep</u>, 2003. http:// parentingteens.about.com.

12. Estés, Clarissa Pinkola, *Women Who Run With the Wolves*. New York: Ballantine Books, 1977, pp. 91-106.

13. Dr. G. Tadorov. <u>Sweat, Skin pH and Acid Mantle</u>. 1998-2001, http://www. smartskincare.com.

14. DeFelice, Joy. *The Effects of Light on the Menstrual Cycle*. Spokan, WA: Sacred Heart Medical Center, 1996.

15. Chamberlain, Sara. <u>Toxic Tampons Pose Health Risks</u>. Earth Island Journal, 1995. http://www.earthisland.org/

16. Masters, William and Virginia Johnson. *Sex and Human Loving*. Boston: Little Brown and Company, 1985, pp. 35-38.

17. Zinn, Howard. *A People's History of the United States*. New York, NY: Harper Collins Publishers, 2003, p. 20.

18. Wolfe, Honora Lee. Menopause, *A Second Spring: Making a Smooth Transition with Traditional Chinese Medicine*. Boulder, CO: Blue Poppy Press, 1992, pp. 81-82.

19. Conway. *Maiden, Mother, Crone*. St. Paul, MN: Llewellyn Publications, 1994, pp. 27-31.

20. Bulfinch, Thomas. *Bulfinch's Mythology. The Age of Chivalry or Legends of King Arthur*. http://www.bulfinch.org.

21. Johnson, Linda. *Daughters of the Goddess: The Women Saints of India*. St. Paul, MN: Yes International Publishers, 1994, pp. 93-94.

22. Ideas for this ritual were taken from *Women's Medicine Ways*, by Marcia Stark.

23. Nofziger, Margaret. *Signs of Fertility, The Personal Science of Natural Birth Control*. Deetsville, Alabama: MND publishing, Inc. 1998, pp. 5-9.

24. The following books give a clear presentation of fertility awareness: *A Cooperative Method of Natural Birth Control* by Margaret Nofziger, *Signs of Fertility* by Margaret Nofziger, *A Couple's Guide to Fertility* by Rose Fuller.

25. Chang, Stephen. *The Tao of Sexology*. Reno, NV: Tao Publishing, 1986, p. 67.

26. Hill, Napoleon. *Think and Grow Rich*. Hollywood, CA: Wilshire Book Company, 1966, pp. 200-219.

28. Information on sexually transmitted disease is available from the Medical Institute for Sexual Health, P.O. Box 162306, Austin, TX, 78716-2306, 800-892-9484, http://www.medinstitute.org.

29. Dr. Michel Odent. *The Scientification of Love*. London/New York: Free Association Books, 1999, p. 94.

30. Balaskas, Janet. *Active Birth, The New Approach to Giving Birth Naturally*. Harvard and Boston, Massachusetts: The Harvard Common Press, 1992, pp. 118-125.

31. La Leche League International, *Womanly Art of Breastfeeding*. Schaumburg, Ill: Published by La Leche League International, 1997, p. 362.

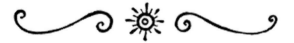

CPSIA information can be obtained at www.ICGtesting.com
Printed in the USA
LVOW032128270512

283474LV00004B/38/P